Telephone Medicine
Triage and Training
A Handbook for Primary Care Health Professionals

Harvey P. Katz, MD

Reprint courtesy of Ross Laboratories, makers of:

•**SIMILAC**® Infant Formulas

•**ISOMIL**® Soy Protein Formulas

•**ALIMENTUM**® Protein Hydrolysate Formula With Iron

D0140379

 F.A. DAVIS COMPANY • **Philadelphia, PA**

Previously published by Slack Incorporated, Thorofare, NJ.

Printed in the United States of America

Last digit indicates print number: 10   9   8   7   6   5   4   3   2

As new scientific information becomes available through basic and clinical research, recommended treatments and drug therapies undergo changes. The author(s) and publisher have done everything possible to make this book accurate, up to date, and in accord with accepted standards at the time of publication. The authors, editors, and publisher are not responsible for errors or omissions or for consequences from application of the book, and make no warranty, expressed or implied, in regard to the contents of the book. Any practice described in this book should be applied by the reader in accordance with professional standards of care used in regard to the unique circumstances that may apply in each situation. The reader is advised always to check product information (package inserts) for changes and new information regarding dose and contraindications before administering any drug. Caution is especially urged when using new or infrequently ordered drugs.

Contents

Foreword

The meager but important literature on the use of the telephone in pediatric practice provides ample justification for this book. Extensive use of the phone in our culture for such diverse purposes as shopping, keeping families together, socializing, and conducting business should have alerted us to the potential of Bell's invention for the provision of medical care. Yet it is virtually ignored in medical education. Household surveys indicate that at least one-fifth of all child contacts with the health care system are by phone. About one-sixth of the average working day in office-based practice is spent on the phone with patients. Phone calls concern children of the same age as those seen face-to-face in pediatric practice: 60% are under age 5 and 80% are under age 10. Ninety percent of callers to office-based practices are regular patients of the pediatrician—the same proportion as those who are encountered in the office. Slightly fewer (60%) of the calls to office-based pediatricians are occasioned by new problems than is the case for office visits. About 30% of telephone calls result in a scheduled face-to-face visit. In contrast to practice, where only 20% of contacts take 5 minutes or less, 90% of phone calls are this short.

Why does the telephone receive so little attention in medical education? Partly because of the meager interest in common everyday problems that afflict patients. Another reason may be the emphasis in medical education on diagnoses that rely heavily on the physical examination or on the performance of laboratory tests and x-rays. Needless to say, both are precluded by telephone contacts.

As with all good medical literature, Dr. Katz's manual sharpens our understanding of the issues. It provides information and skills with which to perform better, and at the same time it raises new questions. Under which circumstances should the use of the phone be encouraged? For adequate care over the phone, is it important that physicians know their patients well? The fact that a greater proportion of phone visits are by "regular" patients than is the case for office patients suggests that telephone calls are used proportionately more when there is an established relationship. When practitioners move into group settings from solo practice settings, their patients make more office visits than previously, most likely because relative unfamiliarity of the other practitioners decreases the extent to which a phone consultation substitutes for a marginally necessary visit.

Is the phone used more under certain payment arrangements than under others? Theoretically, it might be expected that phones would be used in cases where a physician asks for prepayment, in order to avoid unnecessary and costly visits.

Is optimum use of the phone facilitated by prior education of patients and, if so, how can less well-educated patients be helped to make better use of the phone? Studies of the outcome of care given by phone to less well-educated patients as compared with better educated patients, controlling for duration of the practitioner–patient relationship, might improve the effectiveness of phone contacts.

Do studies in which the duration of the practitioner-patient relationship is controlled show that older physicians or those with better training and experience with phone contacts accomplish more through them than younger or less well-trained and less experienced physicians? If so, the mechanisms by which skills in history-taking reduce reliance on the physical examination or laboratory become significant.

Recognition by physicians of concerns expressed by patients is a facet of care that deserves improvement, even in face-to-face contacts. Does experience in handling problems by phone sharpen skills in listening to and heeding patients when they are at hand? If so, skills developed for phone consultation could have spill-over benefit for other types of care.

Does management by phone increase the likelihood of a repeat visit? Merely asking this question makes us realize that we have little information about the number of face-to-face visits that require additional visits because the patient did not improve.

By providing wisdom in critical areas, Dr. Katz has focused our attention on a far broader range of issues that lie at the heart of medical care: the nature of the processes of problem recognition; the relative importance of listening, observing, and testing as tools of diagnosis; the importance of continuity of practitioner; and the receptivity of different types of patients to a more active role in care and the extent of knowledge required to implement it. This is a timely, useful, and provocative book by a thoughtful and eclectic physician.

Barbara H. Starfield, M.D., M.P.H.
Professor and Head
School of Hygiene and Public Health
  and School of Medicine
Health Care Organization
Johns Hopkins University
Baltimore, Maryland

Preface
To Second Edition

Amid the constant bustle of primary care practice there is a sound that seemingly never stops—the ring of the telephone. The cacophony of requests by telephone flowing into our practices has worked its way into the very fabric of medicine today. Acutely ill patients calling for same-day appointments; camp and school physical forms due yesterday; 911 type emergency calls from out of the blue; questions about insurance coverage, shots, the latest medical article's revelation in the local newspaper; routine and follow-up appointments that have to be worked into already overbooked schedules; requests for medical advice and home treatment—an unending and unpredictable current across the lines; an orchestra of thousands of calls daily searching for a score and conductor; at days end (does it ever come)—exhaustion.

Managing the telephone represents one of the great challenges of ambulatory medical practice. In the original 1982 preface of this book, I wrote "One of the strongest links in the chain of communication between patient and physician is the telephone." This has not changed. Never before has the demand for service been greater and the need for better ways to manage the telephone more acute. As some of you may notice, the title of the book has been changed from the *Telephone Manual of Pediatric Care* to *Telephone Medicine: Triage and Training—A Handbook for Primary Care Health Professionals* in order to more accurately describe its contents. The intended audience includes support staff, medical assistants, nurses, nurse practitioners, physician assistants, medical students, housestaff, and the family practitioners and pediatricians who employ and work with these health care professionals. The goal of this edition remains the same, namely to provide a practical approach to telephone medicine triage and training, and to heighten the awareness among health care professionals of the triple impact of the telephone on quality of health care, patient service, and staff satisfaction. The response to the first edition has been very gratifying and has stimulated some new enhancements.

The Handbook is divided into four sections. The first section, The Organization and Art of Telephone Medicine, has been expanded to include an introductory overview of the problems and complexities of the telephone encounter, with a personalized quality of telephone medicine checklist. Several new chapters include: 1) the art of dealing with patients on the telephone, highlighting the need for training in telephone specialty skills; 2) the anatomy of a telephone encounter,

3) guidelines for patients on how to use the telephone more effectively; 4) important medico-legal and risk-management issues; and 5) a practical four-step approach to improving telephone quality and service that can be implemented in any health care setting.

In the second section, Symptoms, Decision Guidelines, and Home Management Advice, for each symptom, a set of questions and decision guidelines has been designed to help distinguish those problems which require an office visit from those that can be safely managed at home. For those problems requiring an appointment, an indication of when the office visit should occur is included, e.g., immediately (emergency), as soon as possible, same session, same day, or a future appointment. Medical advice is included for those problems that can be managed at home. The third section is devoted to the subject of evaluation. Scenarios with a companion checklist are included to help evaluate history taking and decision making by staff to encourage periodic assessment and continuing education in telephone management. The concluding appendix draws attention to potential pitfalls, and presents information relevant to prescribing medication over the phone.

Ideally, the book should be used regularly for both study and as a handy reference. It is important to emphasize that the material in the Handbook is flexible. Individualization is encouraged depending upon the characteristics, clinicians, and staff unique to any given practice or setting. It is my hope that this Handbook will provide a practical, how one-can-do-it framework for those health professionals who play a role on the firing line of telephone medicine and their supervisors, and that it will make our jobs more satisfying, while at the same time accomplishing the common goal of improved quality and service to our patients.

Acknowledgments

Telephone Medicine: Triage and Training—A Handbook for Primary Care Health Professionals and its predecessor, the *Telephone Manual of Pediatric Care* were made possible by the efforts and encouragement of many individuals. I appreciate the suggestions and encouragement of my colleagues and our staff at the Harvard Community Health Plan, and the stimulating health care environment that HCHP provides. My pediatric patients and their parents have contributed more than they know. I am especially grateful for the spirit of cooperation and skills of Ms. Christine Johnson, the first telephone specialist trained with these methods in 1971. Most of all, I thank my wife Marion, Tamara, David, and Tanya for understanding and tolerating the constant ring of the telephone in our home. It has been a particular pleasure to have worked with Marion, whose creative talent as a photographer I admire so greatly.

About the Author

Harvey P. Katz is a Health Center Medical Director at the Harvard Community Health Plan, New England's largest managed health care delivery system, and an Associate Clinical Professor of Pediatrics at the Harvard Medical School. Prior to his move to Boston, Dr. Katz was an Associate Professor of Pediatrics at Johns Hopkins School of Medicine where he started the Columbia Medical Plan, a multispecialty group practice for both prepaid and fee-for-service members, and served as Chief of Pediatrics, Associate Medical Director, and Director of Quality Assurance and Health Education. Dr. Katz completed his pediatric residency training at the Harriett Lane Home of the Johns Hopkins Hospital and a pediatric endocrinology fellowship at the University of California Medical School, San Francisco. Dr. Katz is a member of the American Academy of Pediatrics, the Endocrine Society, and the Lawson Wilkins Pediatric Endocrine Society. He has practiced pediatric medicine for over 25 years. An author of numerous papers and textbook chapters, Dr. Katz has a long-standing interest in the organization and delivery of health care, with an emphasis on quality, efficiency, and effectiveness.

About The Photographer

Belgian-born Marion Mayer Katz is a free-lance photographer known for her sensitive portraits, inspiring landscapes, and creative still lifes. She has studied at the Maryland Institute of Art and the Antioch Visual Arts Center. Ms. Katz's work has been widely exhibited in numerous juried shows in Washington, DC, Maryland, and the Art League in Old Town, Alexandria, Virginia. One such exhibit powerfully portrayed handicapped children and was entitled, "A Different Beauty." Several of Ms. Katz's photographs have been selected for the prestigious art collection of the Federal Reserve Bank of Richmond, VA. Ms. Katz's work was also exhibited as part of the traveling International Photography show in San Francisco, Los Angeles, Dallas, Seattle, and Chicago, and has appeared in several books and photography magazines. Before moving to Boston, she completed a photographic monograph depicting the work of Maryland artists who were awarded grants by the Maryland Arts Council. Marion Katz was the former photography editor of the literary magazine, the *Little Patuxent Review*, and a member of the Visual Arts Alliance of Howard County, MD, and the International Photography Society.

Section I

The Organization and Art of Telephone Medicine

CHAPTER 1

Overview, Complexity, and Opportunity for Quality Improvement

"One afternoon, Mark Twain, who lost more than one hard-earned fortune by investing in hare-brained schemes, described to him in glittering terms, observed a tall, spare man with kindly blue eyes and an eager face coming up the path with a strange contraption under his arm. Yes, it was an invention and the man explained it to the humorist, who listened politely, but said he had been burned too often. 'But I'm not asking you to invest a fortune,' explained the man. You can have as large a share as you want for $500.' Mark Twain shook his head; the invention didn't make sense. The tall, stooped figure started away. 'What did you say your name was?' the author called after him. 'Bell,' replied the inventor a little sadly. 'Alexander Graham Bell.'"

- Vasant Coryell
The Christian Science Monitor - circa 1876

"Today the ringing of the telephone takes precedence over everything. It reaches a point of terrorism, particularly at dinnertime."

- Neils Diffrient
The New York Times - December 16, 1986

On March 7, 1876, the first telephone patent (No. 174,465) was issued to a Mark Twain-spurned inventor and professor of vocal physiology at Boston University.[1] Professor Bell would no doubt have been incredulous at the prediction that 100 years later, there would be 153 million telephones in the United States,[2] along with terms like PBX (private branch exchange), Centrex, BOC (Bell operating companies), ACD (automatic call distribution), voice mailboxes, and cellular phones. Nor could physicians of that day dream how profoundly the telephone would impact upon the practice of medicine.

While Bell's invention has become an indispensable communication link between physicians and patients, the telephone has also become a focal point of patient complaints about poor service ("May I place you on 'hold?'—CLICK), and a major cause of dissatisfaction among clinicians and their medical support staff. In one study, 36% of physicians reported the telephone as their greatest practice problem.[3] This is probably understated. It was not unexpected that 54% of after-midnight calls were deemed inappropriate by pediatricians.[4]

Problems within telephone medicine segregate into three general categories: 1) volume overload with access difficulties; 2) the stress on clinicians of nonemergency nighttime calls; and 3) a myriad of issues relating to office telephone triage—what should be delegated and to whom, namely, who's responsible for what? Volume overload has been documented in several studies. The telephone may consume up to 30% of total practice time for some primary care physicians.[5] In one busy primary care practice of six clinicians, 1000 calls daily, 100 occurring hourly during the busiest hours of the day, and an average of one new ring every 90 seconds is not unusual.[6] Since there is never advance warning as to the calls' content, the receiver must be especially well-trained and integrated into the office systems through his or her role on the telephone. All too frequently, through no fault of the support staff, this is not the case, and the endpoint of the telephone encounter is either frustration or error. The quality of telephone medicine is a challenge facing not only primary care, but all of the medical and surgical specialties as well.

Since it is impossible for the physician to speak to every patient who calls, the delegation of some degree of telephone responsibility is inevitable. It is no surprise, therefore, that the telephone has emerged as a serious medico-legal threat. A Midwest jury recently awarded $2.5 million to a family who claimed that there was a delay in the diagnosis of their daughter's meningitis, specifically because of telephone advice the parents received from the office nurse. This registered nurse was a member of a well-trained nurse telephone counseling staff employed by a highly respected pediatric group. The jury concluded that, while the nurse's counseling service was acceptable, she failed to follow established guidelines.[7]

The role and management of the telephone in medicine, given its import and complexity, deserves more attention than it receives. The purpose of this introduction is threefold: to highlight the results of a telephone medicine satisfaction survey among pediatric department heads; to emphasize the complexity and interplay of the multiple factors influencing the quality of telephone medicine satisfaction survey among pediatric department heads; to emphasize the complexity and interplay of the multiple factors influencing the quality of telephone medicine; and to stress the importance of training in telephone management as one part of the overall strategy to improve the quality of office telephone management and triage.

4

In 1987, a national survey was conducted to determine the level of satisfaction with the process of telephone medicine.[8] A survey among HMO chiefs was stimulated by an earlier finding that 42% of fee-for-service pediatricians in Denver and Baltimore were dissatisfied with the telephone aspect of their practice.[9] The HMO survey included both group and staff models; 67 of 123 pediatric chiefs responded to the questionnaire (54%). Of the 67 respondents, 45% reported telephone dissatisfaction within their departments, indicating feelings identical to their fee-for-service counterparts. The number of calls per day, evening, and weekend between the fee-for-service and the HMO practices were comparable. In the HMO sample[8], only 56% of the pediatric departments provided their staff with regularly scheduled in-service teaching in telephone management skills. Dissatisfied chiefs were less likely to delegate or document calls, and they cited improved staff training and decreased delays in response time to patient calls as the improvements that were most needed. Satisfied chiefs remarked that the best features of their telephone system were their excellent staff and how promptly they were able to respond to patient calls. Although there was no attempt to measure patient and staff satisfaction in this survey, patients and medical support staff alike often rank the telephone as their major problem.

As complicated as a face-to-face patient encounter may be, a telephone encounter is even more complex. There is less time, no body language, and rarely is there an opportunity for second thoughts once the call is over and the receiver goes on to the next call. In the heat of a hectic day, we frequently lose sight of the complexity of the multiple variables that influence a single telephone encounter. These variables include: 1) the patient; 2) the skill and preparation of the staff and the supports given to them; 3) the system in which they work, 4) the nature of the call, and 5) the medico-legal issues within the system. The interplay of these multiple factors is illustrated in the fishbone, or Ishikawa cause-and-effect diagram (Figure 1). It is the intertwining of these multiple factors that determines the outcome of every telephone encounter. Each piece of the Ishikawa diagram represents a process. Although training and the preparation of support staff in telephone skills is only one process in the system, its importance surfaces in all of the categories.

Given the complexity of the system and the often overwhelming volume of telephone calls in American health care, it is no wonder that the lowly telephone has become public enemy number one. Where to start to solve some of the problems? If our goal is to improve quality and service, lessons may be learned from the Theory of Continuous Improvement,[10] which is based on understanding each small process that makes up the larger systems. Slow revisions of small pieces of

Figure 1

Ishikawa Cause and Effect Diagram

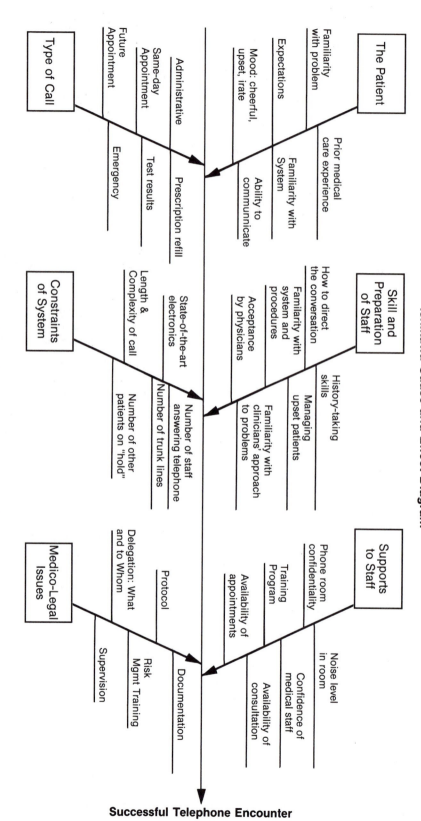

Fishbone Diagram illustrating the interplay of Variables or inputs which determine a desired outcome

the process, based on sound data and clarification of the root defect in a process, leads to a continuing cycle of improvement. The shift is away from our current focus on problems and people, to identifying, understanding, and then acting on processes in need of improvement. Although the worlds of medicine and industry are different, there are common themes and lessons to be learned from quality control theorists like Deming,[11] and Juran,[12] who are credited with quality improvement methods successfully used in Japan and in a growing number of U.S. organizations.

How well do we really prepare our medical support staff for this critical office responsibility—and how prepared are we as their supervisors?[13] Just because someone answers the phone, there is often the assumption that the person will automatically know what to do. In a 1986 survey of 151 pediatric residency programs, only 45% offered any specific training in telephone medicine.[14] The residents were managing an average of 19 calls daily; only half of the programs documented any phone calls. The ambulatory care setting and our medical offices provide an excellent environment for such training, which can include a variety of teaching methods for our staff, such as mock role-playing and the critiquing of live tapes and video-script scenarios of telephone encounters as springboards for group discussions of telephone management protocols. The importance of patient and parent education in all areas of telephone use in the evaluation and reporting of their problems cannot be overemphasized. Instructions in telephone use for our patients should be explicit, as illustrated in Chapter 7.

The importance of the telephone in our practices can be personalized with a telephone quality-of-care checklist (Table 1). Score one point for each YES. If any clinician's score is close to 12, hearty congratulations! If there is room for the Theory of Continuous Improvement, it would seem that the lowly telephone should demand as much time in our practices as any other high-tech aspect. As one way to get started, a four-step process is detailed in Chapter 10. These include: 1) getting to know your own system better, 2) a period of study for all staff, 3) a method by which staff can train other staff more effectively, and 4) an increased level of involvement by clinicians in evaluating the performance and skill level of those on our staff who answer the phone. Our common goals are improved quality of care, service, and both staff and patient satisfaction.

Table 1
Telephone Quality of Care Checklist

1. Do you know how many phone calls your office receives daily, and what are the top six reasons for calls?   YES   NO
2. Is the average duration of employment for your office telephone staff greater than two years?   YES   NO
3. Have you recruited the right person for the job?   YES   NO
4. Do you have a formalized training of telephone management/triage in your office practice?   YES   NO
5. Do you have written protocols, specific guidelines, and office procedures for your staff?   YES   NO
6. Do you have written protocols for emergencies and for what to do when physicians are not in the office?   YES   NO
7. Do you document all medically significant phone calls?   YES   NO
8. Do you write smarter rather than longer?   YES   NO
9. Does your staff have a low threshold to bring patients in for an office visit?   YES   NO
10. Have you received no complaints from patients about the telephone or telephone staff in the last month?   YES   NO
11. Do you personally review telephone procedures regularly with your staff to be sure that only conditions that are appropriate for management by telephone are so managed?   YES   NO
12. Have you met with your staff in the last two months to talk about the telephone and to listen to their problems?   YES   NO

REFERENCES

1. Bell AG: Researches in telephony. Proc Amer Acad Arts and Sciences 1876; 12:1-10.
2. The Telephone. Collier's Encyclopedia, Macmillan Educational Corp, New York, 1979; 22:121-133.
3. Deisher RW, Berby AJ, Sturman MJ: Changing trends in pediatric practice. Pediatrics 1960; 25:711-716.
4. Caplan S, Orr S, Skulstad J, et al: After hours telephone use in urban pediatric primary care centers. A M J Dis Child 1983; 137:879-882.
5. Hessel SJ, Haggerty RJ: General Pediatrics: A study of practice in mid-1960's. J Pediatrics 1968; 73:271-279.

6. Katz HP, unpublished data.

7. Katz HP and Wick W: Telephone medicine—the Newest Medico-Legal Threat. Presentation to Council on Pediatric Practice. Annual meeting, AAP, 1989.

8. Fosarelli P and Katz HP: Residents on the phone. Letters to the editor. Pediatrics 1987; 79:311-312.

9. Fosarelli P and Schmitt D: Telephone dissatisfaction in pediatric practice: Denver and Baltimore. Pediatrics 1987; 80:28-31.

10. Berwick D: Continuous improvement as an ideal in health care. Sounding board. New Eng J Med, 1989; 320:53-56.

11. Deming WE: Out of the Crisis. Cambridge, Massachusetts Institute of Technology. Center for Advanced Engineering Study, 1986.

12. Juran JM: Managerial Breakthrough, New York, McGraw-Hill Co., 1964.

13. Fosarelli PD: The emphasis of telephone medicine in pediatric training programs. Am J Dis Child 1985; 139:555-557.

14. Wood PR: Pediatric resident training in telephone management: a survey of training programs in the United States 1986; 77:822-825.

CHAPTER **2**

Role of the Telephone in Medical Care and Comprehensive Bibliography of Telephone Medicine Literature

In the year of the discovery of the telephone, 1876, the inventor, Alexander Graham Bell, and his assistant, Tom Watson, sold approximately 1,000 telephones. One year after, 10,000 people were using the telephone, while 100 years later, telephones had found their way into more than 153 million homes in the United States. Although the telephone is ubiquitous in the health care system, it has only been in the past 5 years that increased interest has been shown in studying and exploring its potential in ambulatory care settings. Before this time, little attention was paid to this communication medium despite the fact that 13 percent of all patient care contacts in the United States, and 30 percent for pediatricians, are by telephone. The dependence of both patients and physicians on this medium has been documented in several time-motion studies and medical care surveys, which have delineated those factors that influence telephone care behavior, such as socioeconomic status, age, and type of illness.

With few exceptions, the specific details of the delegation of telephone care responsibility to nonphysicians, although quite acceptable to parents, have not been well defined. This is unfortunate, since an unstructured setting encourages the assumption of more management responsibilities than physicians perceive they actually delegate. Marginally trained personnel in offices, clinics, and answering services may advise, appoint, and refer patients according to vague guidelines, potentially generating unnecessary visits or delaying essential care. Several investigators, studying telephone care process with provider-blind mock encounters, detected significant deficiencies in history taking, accuracy of advice, and communication style by house officers, health associates, and even physicians who were not specifically trained in telephone care. Conversely, few decision errors and a high level of parental acceptance have been found in nursing personnel who were trained for a telephone care role. A problem has been that allied health professionals may experience dissatisfaction with a predominantly telephone care responsibility that leaves little time for direct patient care and nursing.

Within pediatrics and family practice, the telephone has been used as an aid in physical diagnoses, in poison control centers, as a link to subspecialty consultation from rural areas, as a hotline for parents to obtain throat culture results, and by pediatric triage nurses in an inner city emergency room. The use and evaluation of nonnursing personnel in telephone triage and management has only recently been tested, by means of both process and outcome measures of quality of care, with positive results. These findings offer reassurance to those who might choose to delegate this responsibility to either nursing or nonnursing personnel under physician supervision, since it appears that it is possible to design a cost-effective telephone system using personnel with special training to effectively and safely sort out and advise the large number of minor problems that are commonly presented by telephone in pediatric and family practice, with the maintenance of high levels of parental satisfaction and acceptance. Issues such as the health education value of telephone advice, the impact upon health care utilization, and the most effective methods for training housestaff are ripe subjects for future exploration.

COMPREHENSIVE TELEPHONE CARE BIBLIOGRAPHY AND CHRONOLOGY

Bell AG: Researches in Telephony. *Proc Amer Acad Arts and Sciences* 1876; 12:1–10.

Deisher RW, Berby AJ, Sturman MJ. Changing Trends in Pediatric Practice. *Pediatrics* 1960; 25:711–716.

Aldrich RH: *Careers in Pediatrics*, Report of the thirty-sixth Ross Conference of pediatric research. 1960.

Bergman AB, Dassel SW, Wedgewood RJ: Time-motion study of practicing pediatrics. *Pediatrics* 1966; 38:254.

Hessel SJ, Haggerty RJ: A study of practice in the mid-1960's. *J Pediatr* 1968; 73:271–279.

Hessel SJ, Haggerty RJ: General Pediatrics: A study of practice in the mid-1960s. *J Pediatr* 1968; 73:271–279.

Heagarty MC, Robertson L, Kosa J, et al: Use of the telephone by low-income families. *J Pediatr* 1968; 73:740–744.

Heagarty M: The use of the telephone in pediatric practice, in Green M, Heagarty R (eds): *Ambulatory Pediatrics.* Philadelphia, WB Saunders Co, 1968; pp 136–139.

Patterson P, Bergman A: Time motion study of six pediatric office assistants. *N Eng J Med* 1969; 281:771–774.

Patterson P, Bergman A, Wedgewood R: Parent reaction to the concept of pediatric assistants. *Pediatrics* 1969; 44:69–75.

Hercules C, Charney E: Availability and attentiveness—Are these compatible in pediatric practice. *Clin Pediatr* 1969; 8:381–388.

Charney E, Kitzman H: The child-health nurse (pediatric nurse practitioner) in private practice—A controlled trial. *N Eng J Med* 1971; 285:1353–1358.

Katz HP: Telephone utilization in a prepaid multispecialty group practice. Eleventh Annual Meeting, Abstracts of the Ambulatory Pediatric Association meetings, 1971, p 42.

Silver H, Duncan B: Time-motion study of pediatric nurse practitioners: Comparison with "regular" office nurses and pediatricians. *J Pediatr* 1971; 79:331–336.

Pope CR, Yoshioka SS, Greenlick MR: Determinants of medical care utilization—The use of the telephone for reporting symptoms. *J Health Soc Behav* 1971; 12:155–162.

Strain J, Miller J: The preparation, utilization and evaluation of a registered nurse trained to give telephone advice in a private pediatric office. *Pediatrics* 1971; 47:1051–1056.

Tripp S: Telephone Techniques in Pediatric Practice. *Am J Nursing* 1971; 71:1722–1724.

Reece RM, Robertson LS, Alpert II: The telephone answering service—A survey of use by general practitioners and pediatricians in Massachusetts. *Clin Pediatr* 1972; 11:40–43.

Greenlick MR, Freeborn DK, Colombo TJ: Comparing the use of medical services by a medically indigent and a general membership population in a comprehensive prepaid group practice program. *Med Care* 1972; 10(3):187–200.

Greenlick MR, Freeborn DK, Gambill GL, et al: Determinants of medical care utilization—The role of the telephone in total medical care. *Med Care* 1973; 11(2):121–134.

Katz HP, Katz J, Bernstein M, et al: Night call—An extended role for the nurse practitioner. Fourteenth Annual Meeting, Abstracts of the Ambulatory Pediatric Association meetings, 1974, p 70.

Ott JE, Bellaire J, Machota P, et al: Patient management by telephone by child health associates and pediatric house officers. *J Med Educ* 1974; 49:596–600.

Brown SB, Eberle BJ: Use of telephone by pediatric house staff—A technique for pediatric care not taught. *J Pediatr* 1974; 84:117–120. 1974.

Arnold R: How does a pediatrician spend his time? *Clin Pediatr* 1975; 12:611.

Katz HP, Mushlin A, Posen J: Quality of telephone care: Assessment of a system utilizing non-physician personnel. *Am J Public Health* 1978; 68:31.

Perrin EC, Goodman HC: Telephone management of acute pediatric illnesses. *N Eng J Med* 1978; 298:130–135.

Rosekrans J, Limbo D, Kaplan D, et al: *Pediatric Telephone Protocols*, Darien, Conn, Patient Care Publications, Inc, 1979.

Levy JC, Rosekrans J, Lamb GA, et al: Development and field testing of protocols for the management of pediatric telephone calls: Protocols for pediatric telephone calls. *Pediatrics* 1979; 64:558–563.

Strasser PH, Levy JC, Lamb GA, et al: Controlled clinical trial of pediatric telephone protocols. *Pediatrics* 1979; 64:553–557.

Schmitt BD: *Pediatric Telephone Advice*, Boston, Little, Brown & Co, 1980.

Brown JL: *Telephone Medicine*, St Louis, C.V. Mosby Co, 1980.

Caplan S, Orr S, Skulstad J, et al: After hours telephone use in urban pediatric primary care centers.*AMJ Dis Child* 1983; 137:879–882.

Fosarelli PD: The emphasis of telephone medicine in pediatric training programs. *AMJ Dis Child* 1985; 139:555–557.

Wood PR: Pediatric resident training in telephone management: a survey of training programs in the United States 1986; 77:822–825.

Fosarelli P and Katz HP: Residents on the Phone. Letters to the Editor. *Pediatrics* 1987; 79:311–312.

Fosarelli P and Schmitt D: Telephone Dissatisfaction in Pediatric Practice: Denver and Baltimore. *Pediatrics* 1987; 80:28–31.

Katz HP and Wick W: Telephone Medicine—the Newest Medico-Legal Threat. Presentation to Council on Pediatric Practice. Annual meeting, AAP, 1989.

Wood PR, Littlefield JH, and Foulds DM: Telephone Management Curriculum for Pediatric Interns: A Controlled Trial. *Pediatrics* 1989; 83:925–930.

CHAPTER **3**

Organizing a Total Telephone Care System Within an Office or Clinic

A time honored, traditional approach to providing telephone care by practitioners has been to start off each day with a *phone hour,* either at the office or home. The personal touch of this method has been its greatest strength and it remains popular among many patients and physicians. However, there are a number of drawbacks. There are more patients who wish to speak with their physician than there is time to respond; a few patients can monopolize the majority of time causing a backlog of calls; patients still need to call at other times during the day; and many of the calls really do not require a physician. Thus, even a successful phone hour needs to be supplemented by telephone care for the remainder of the day. The personal touch can be preserved even if the physician delegates this responsibility to others. Both conceptually (for purposes of organizing training of new personnel) as well as organizationally (if the practice or clinic is large enough to justify multiple phones), it may be helpful to view the function of a telephone care system as a two-part unit, administrative information consisting mainly of *future appointments* and *problem care* (Fig. 2).

FUTURE APPOINTMENTS

The separation of future appointments from other telephone calls in a busy office decreases telephone congestion and provides a quicker response. Once the number and type of phone calls in any given medical practice have been analyzed, a practitioner (with help from the telephone company if requested) can decide whether it would be feasible to have a separate telephone number for future appointments and immediate telephone care (Fig. 2). In a small practice where all telephone calls enter via one line, the distinction between the two units is more a conceptual one, which should assist in training and orienting new personnel. Staff should be trained in making future appointments according to specific guidelines (Table 2), which indicate the time allocation for specific prob-

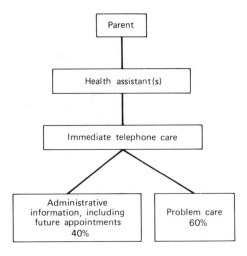

Figure 2

Organization of telephone care system into components of administrative information, including future appointments and problem care. Depending on the size of the practice, two or more health assistants with separate lines of responsibility will be needed. All telephone assistants should be cross-trained so that they can handle each component.

lems. The skill in implementing these guidelines is critical to the success of the program. It is also helpful for staff to view the timing of appointments (Table 3) in relation to the presenting complaint, namely, whether the call is a true emergency, or whether the problem warrants an appointment immediately, later the same day, or in the near future (within 2 weeks at most). Families should be instructed to call for future appointments outside the times of peak phone calls (after 10 A.M. and before 4 P.M.) in order to avoid the rush of calls reporting illness complaints early in the morning and after school. One or more office personnel can staff the future and immediate telephone care telephone lines, depending on the volume of calls (e.g., two or three people may be needed from 8:30 A.M. to 10 A.M., and then only one or two for the remainder of the day). As a point of reference, between 250 and 350 phone calls per day can be managed efficiently in such a system. It is estimated that approximately two-thirds of calls will be for problem care and the remainder for future appointments and other administrative information, such as prescription refills, requests for laboratory results, school and camp forms, and other miscellaneous items.

Table 2

GUIDELINES AND DESCRIPTIONS FOR FUTURE APPOINTMENTS

Health Care Provider	Sample Allocations	Column for Individual Differences
Pediatrician/Family Practitioner		
New patient	30 min	
New patient with medical problem	45 min	
Follow-up health review and physical examination		
Well baby 2 mos–18 mos	15 min	
$2\frac{1}{2}$ yr–17 yr	15–30 min	
2-wk first well baby visit	30 min	
Established patient with a medical problem	30 min	
Follow-up of a chronic problem	30 min	
Same day appointments—acute care	15 min	
Pediatric or Family Nurse Practitioner		
New patient	30–45 min	
New family with two children	1 hr 15 min	
2-wk first well baby visit	30–45 min	
Pediatric Nurse Practitioner		
Follow-up well baby visit	15–30 min	
Same day appointments—acute care	15 min	
Specialty Problems		
Endocrine		
New patient	1 hr	
Follow-up	30 min	
Renal clinic	1 hr	
Neurology clinic	1 hr	
Learning disability and behavior problems	1 hr 15 min	
Other (fill in as needed)		

Table 3
APPOINTMENT MAKING IN RELATION TO PRESENTING COMPLAINT[a]

Emergencies (life-threatening illness)

Acute allergic reaction with respiratory difficulty

Convulsion

Overdose of medication

Diabetic reaction

Poisoning

Coma or unconsciousness

Uncontrollable bleeding

Drowning or near drowning

Penetrating wounds of stomach or chest

Behavior change following head trauma

Immediate Appointment

Acting very ill (very irritable or lethargic)

Sudden change in any condition and symptoms worsening

Difficulty breathing and/or asthma attack

Possible fracture

Convulsion that has stopped and child now acting well

Severe abdominal pain or pain localized to the right lower abdomen

Acute allergic reactions without respiratory symptoms

Extremely anxious parent

Fall from high place

Forceful and repetitive vomiting

Paralysis or weakness of a limb

Head trauma

Severe pain of any type

Stiff neck and ill appearance

Same Day or Same Session (depending upon severity) Appointment.

Earache

Rash

Temperature uncontrolled by treatment

Diarrhea

Stiff neck with muscle strain

Sore throat

Swollen glands

Skin infection, boils

Pain or burning on urination

Symptoms not improving

Table 3 (continued)

Same Day Appointment (continued)

Abdominal pain

Thirst, excessive urinating, hunger, and weight loss (immediate appointment if symptoms severe)

Joint pain or swelling

Future Appointment (soon—1 to 2 days; later—1 to 2 weeks).

Emotional or behavioral problems

School problems

Growth problems

Diagnostic problems with nonacute symptoms that have been present for a long time: headache, enuresis, abdominal pain.

Other diagnostic problems and follow-ups as indicated according to individual physician's guidelines.

[a] The specifics should be modified according to the physician's preferences. Patients are very reluctant to wait so that *whenever possible, there should be an attempt made to give the appointment as quickly as possible,* depending on the time available, as well as the nature of the problem.

PROBLEM CARE

The telephone assistant who receives a non-emergency request for problem care must make one of three basic decisions: (1) whether to schedule an appointment for the same day, (2) to advise in home management, or (3) to refer the telephone call elsewhere (Fig. 3).

Until recently there was very little objective data that could be used to describe the content of telephone care in pediatric practice. The first critical study of telephone care utilization examined the content of all telephone calls received within a busy group practice over a period of 4 weeks. During the study period there were 2,520 telephone encounters

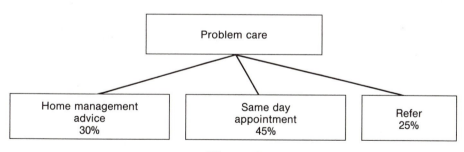

Figure 3

Systems approach to decision-making for telephone calls requesting assistance for health related problems.

Table 4
DISPOSITION AND FREQUENCY DISTRIBUTION OF ILLNESS COMPLAINTS REPORTED BY TELEPHONE

Type of Complaint	Number of Calls	Immediate Visit (%)	Advised for Home Care (%)	Referred to a Pediatrician (%)
Respiratory	620	65	22	5
Gastrointestinal	160	27	60	24
Dermatologic	146	39	45	15
Other[a]	559	42	26	40
Total	1,485	43	38	21

[a]Includes trauma, headache, and symptoms related to the eye, musculoskeletal and genitourinary systems.

during clinic office hours and 516 on evenings and weekends. The three most common acute medical complaints that caused parents to request immediate care were respiratory, gastrointestinal, and skin problems, collectively accounting for 62 percent of all 1,485 illness-related complaints. This data served as a guide to the structure of our training manual. The study also analyzed the frequency distribution of all illness-related complaints according to the decisions made by the telephone care assistants (immediate office appointment versus home management advice) who, in this case, were nonnursing support staff with on-the-job training

Table 5
DISPOSITION FOR IMMEDIATE PROBLEM CARE CALLS

Decision	Total Problem Care Calls (%)
Same day appointment given	45
Advised home management in lieu of appointment	30
Call referred to	25
Pediatrician (10)	
Nurse practitioner (8)	
Future appointments (2)	
Emergency room (2)	
Other department (3)	
Total percent	100
Total number of calls analyzed	1,500

(Table 4). As can be seen, 60 percent of gastrointestinal complaints were managed independently by home advice compared to only 22 percent of respiratory complaints. The study also revealed that significantly more home management advice was given for older children than for infants. Analysis of after-hours data indicated that true emergencies were very rare and that over 90 percent of calls could be managed effectively by both physicians and nurse practitioners with home management advice. While most evening and night telephone calls are received by the physician, an increasing number of practices and clinics are using nurse practitioners or physician assistants to help in this responsibility.

How often a decision is made to advise or appoint by a health care provider depends on a number of factors. These include the training the skill of the provider, to what extent the responsibility to advise is delegated by the supervising physician, how well known a patient and medical history is to be the practice, and the exceptions of the parent. In one setting where decision-making was studied—a balanced health maintenance organization (HMO), fee-for-service practice—it was determined that one-third of calls presenting a medical complaint were advised independently (Table 5). A follow-up of those patients revealed no residual problems and a high degree of parental satisfaction with the instructions and interest shown by the telephone assistant who managed the illness.

Emergencies

While the medical management of emergencies is beyond the scope of this book, the telephone management of an emergency situation could not be more relevant or critical. A potential life or death emergency situation can be lurking behind every routine telephone call. The telephone assistant must be prepared to manage such calls and make important decisions, even in rare instances when the clinicians may be absent from the office. For training and triage purposes the following recommendations are made:

- Those who have a telephone medicine responsibility should review with the supervising physician how potential emergency situations that present by telephone should be managed (see decision guidelines for immediate appointments in Section II and Appendix A: Avoiding Potential Pitfalls. There should be specific instructions about about what to do when the physician may not be immediately available i.e., calling 911 or making arrangements at the nearest local emergency room.
- Whenever there is doubt about a possible emergency situation, the physician should be interrupted immediately. Written protocols should be available and individualized to meet the preference and needs of the practice and supervising physician(s).

- The patient's name and phone number should be obtained early in the conversation, if at all possible, in the event he or she is cut-off. The more informed we are about questions to ask and procedures to follow, the easier it will be to stay calm and mentally alert when an emergency situation arises.

CHAPTER **4**

Telephone Style: Your Voice Creates an Image

The members of the office or clinic staff who are selected for a telephone care responsibility represent the vital link between families and physician. How well this responsibility is performed will determine the way in which patients enter the system, and will have a profound influence on quality of care, patient and physician satisfaction, and the growth of a given medical practice. For these reasons, the individuals recruited for the telephone care position must be carefully selected and properly oriented from the very beginning. The telephone care responsibility should be discussed in detail during the applicant's interview. The individual who is selected is, in effect, the image and voice of the practice, and the wrong person or personality in this sensitive position can spell disaster. As stated previously, the person selected and her background will vary with the medical environment, and should be chosen by the physician or nurse who will assume the full responsibility for the delegation of this function. In most settings, a nurse or nurse practitioner is selected. A potential problem with this arrangement is that a nurse may start with enthusiasm, but become dissatisfied in time, feeling that too much time on the phone detracts from her role in direct patient care. In addition to nurses, many physicians have used a specially trained, nonnurse health assistant. The qualifications for this position include (1) having raised children, (2) intelligence, (3) warmth and compassion, (4) a calm personality, and (5) sound judgment. Although prior medical training is very helpful, it has not been an absolute requirement since structured on-the-job training has proved successful. How much teaching and supervision is necessary depends on the degree of responsibility the practitioner wishes to delegate; the knowledge, experience, motivation, and style of the telephone receptionist; and the characteristics of the population served. A quality assessment of one such system indicated that health assistants effectively and safely advised parents in the home management of a wide variety of medical problems, increasing pediatrician and nurse time for direct contact with patients. The study revealed a high degree of parental satisfaction, and it was felt that the personal approach to medical care was not compromised.

The following paragraph is written as a message to anyone assigned the responsibility of answering the telephone in a medical office. It would be a good idea for those who answer the telephone in a doctor's office to take the time to be recorded and to listen to yourself speaking with patients. The telephone company may provide this service in their traveling training program.

Did you ever stop to think that when you use the telephone, *your voice is you*? And that you and your voice create the image of the office practice that is conveyed to patients. The patient who calls cannot *see* the rest of the staff, modern equipment, or attractive features of the office. It is your voice that creates the visual picture. Your warmth goes a long way in helping patients get better quickly and helps convey that all-important ingredient in medical practice—*caring*. Personality and individual style influence the visual picture. Here are some helpful hints:

- Be alert, wide awake, and always express interest in the caller.
- Send along a friendly smile and greeting with your message.
- Speak clearly, distinctly, and confidently.
- At all times, be polite, warm, and businesslike.
- Go out of your way to be helpful. Put yourself in the patient's shoes.
- Be expressive and put the punctuation into your voice—the ??? and the !!!
- Talk naturally. Use a normal tone of voice and a moderate rate of speech. Avoid slang, technical language, and irrelevant, personal chit-chat. Other patients are waiting. Make every effort to be efficient and relevant so that you can get to other calls quickly.

Patients are quick to sense the desire to help, and if combined with sound, intelligent advice, even the most difficult patient will be understanding and cooperative. If the conversation starts off on the right foot, it will conclude to everyone's satisfaction. If the patient is upset and angry, don't react. If necessary, transfer the call to the physician, along with all available background information. Don't argue with patients. The art of managing an upset patient is discussed in chapter 6. Other helpful suggestions are as follows:

- Answer the phone promptly. Ringing telephones are a source of irritation to everyone. Set a goal of picking up the phone after no more than three rings and make every effort to meet that standard.
- Never give a patient a hard time. If you cannot provide information, offer to find someone who can. When you are overloaded, there is always the useful option of taking down the number and calling back.
- Be discreet, confidential, and sensitive to the problem. When a patient is upset, there is always a reason but you may not know it. For example, there may have been a recent death in the family, or the parent may have been up all night.

- Avoid the "May I put you on hold?" habit. Think how you would feel if the first thing you heard was "Is this an emergency or may I please put you on hold?" and you are on hold before you even have a chance to respond. If you must leave the caller for a moment, explain and ask him or her to wait. "Will you hold the line please while I check that information . . . or while I answer another telephone . . . or while I get the doctor?" If it takes more than a minute, offer to call back if you can. When you do return to the line after a hold, thank the caller for waiting.

This is all basic information that, in the heat of a busy day, may be forgotten. We are all human. Some need more reminders than others. To see how you rate, try evaluating yourself by answering the following questions. If your score is high, then you are well suited for a telephone.

WHAT'S YOUR COURTESY QUOTIENT?

1. Do you answer promptly and greet callers pleasantly? Do you put "good morning" and "thank you for calling" into your voice?
2. Do you identify yourself properly and show that you will take responsibility for the call?
3. Do you use the caller's name and give your full attention to the call?
4. Do you take notes to avoid having your caller repeat information?
5. If you are unable to help a caller, do you explain that you are leaving the line or transferring the call?
6. Do you apologize for delays?
7. Every person who calls you considers his or her call important (or else he wouldn't have made it). Do you handle it that way—as if it were a good friend or close relative?
8. When you promise a callback, do you follow through?
9. Do you place calls as courteously and efficiently as you like to receive them?

CHAPTER **5**

Anatomy of a Telephone Encounter

The telephone encounter, while complex, as described in the Ishikawa cause-and-effect diagram in Chapter 1, has an anatomy of three basic parts:

1. Greeting or "verbal handshake."
2. Obtaining the history or relevant information.
3. Closure by making a disposition or offering help.

The greeting sets the tone for the encounter and is the verbal handshake, pleasant and professional. The greeting should include four points:

1. A friendly introduction, such as "good morning."
2. Name—"This is Ms. Johnson."
3. Identification of the department to make sure callers know they are in the right place—"department of . . ."
4. An offer of help—"may I help you."

Ideally all four points should be used, but when the phone gets too busy, the four points can be abbreviated to save time. Telephone assistants should practice tone and style using a tape recorder to achieve a greeting that comes across as professional and caring. There is a big difference between, "Good morning, this is Chris, may I be of help?" versus "Hello, Pediatrics." Also, try practicing the greeting with erect posture versus slouching with face held downward, and with and without a smile in your voice. Note the difference. Good posture and the appropriate affect create a communication style that helps establish rapport with the patient, which is necessary for eliciting an accurate history.

The second part, obtaining the information that is necessary for a relevant disposition, requires skill in history taking (See Chapter 8), experience, and concentration. Speaking to patients on the telephone is much more difficult than doing so face-to-face. The pace is faster, visual clues are absent, and distractions are all around us—noise, patient traffic, and others asking us to do things in the middle of a conversation. The telephone assistant has to rely on tone and expression, how messages are phrased, and a careful choice of words. Close-ended questions should be used whenever appropriate, "we have appointments available at 2 and 7 p.m., which would be more convenient for you?" works better than "Would you like to come in this afternoon or evening?" and saves time. However, patients should be permitted to express their concerns. Although this takes more time, it is important for an accurate history. The experienced telephone assistant can get to the point quickly by combining an assertive style, being well-informed and professional, and know when to ask closed versus open questions.

The third part of a telephone encounter is coming to closure by offering help. There are three basic types of disposition:

- Give an appointment.
- Take a message for someone else.
- Refer to another source, such as another department, person, specialty area, or local emergency room.

Once the decision and disposition have been made, or you have made an offer to help solve a problem, all efforts should be made to follow through and honor the offer. For example, if the disposition is for someone to call back within an hour, someone should do so. This relies not only upon the telephone assistant staff, but also requires a smooth functioning office message system and the cooperation of all clinicians.

CHAPTER **6**

Guide to
Managing the Upset
or Angry Patient

The ultimate challenge to the telephone medicine specialist is managing an irate, upset patient. Fortunately, this occurs only rarely. However, when it does, the experience can be devastating to the inexperienced telephone assistant who, while trying his or her best to help, finds the encounter out of control. Training and advance preparation for managing this specific type of problem are essential. If you can complete a telephone encounter of this third kind keeping your cool, separating the person from the situation, solving the problem, and turning the angry patient into a loyal and appreciative friend, you truly have mastered the art of telephone medicine. Here are eight helpful tips.

1.   DON'T TAKE IT PERSONALLY.
Contrary to how it feels, the patient's anger is not directed at you personally. The upset patient is angry at the situation over which he or she feels they have no control. It takes training and experience to stay calm, listen and resist the reflex to react.

2.   LET THE PATIENT VENT
Even though it takes time, nothing we say sinks in while an angry patient is blowing off steam. "Hang out like the fog" and wait for the right opening. It always comes, sooner or later, and when it does, grab it out of the air. Anything that sounds positive is a great time to break in. For example, when a patient says, "I can't understand what is going on, I always used to be given an appointment sooner." At that moment the patient is thinking of a more positive experience from the past and is ready to listen.

3.   ACKNOWLEDGE FEELINGS
Establish rapport by using the technique of mirroring feelings. Listen for the pause or a break in the anger and then say, "I don't blame you for feeling that way...specifically, how can I help you" (to mirror means paraphrasing in your own words how the person is feeling).

4. SEPARATE THE PERSON FROM THE SITUATION

This will help you avoid the accuse...defend...reaccuse cycle. A patient says, "You told me the Doctor would call"...followed by the assistant who answers, "No I didn't... and back again to "Yes you most certainly did"...without ever discussing the issue at hand. Although it is difficult, always try to keep the central problem of the call in focus.

5. REFER THE CALL

If you are getting nowhere, or if the call is consuming too much time while other patients are waiting, don't hesitate to ask your supervisor or the patient's clinician to help by speaking to the patient directly. Tell the patient that you will have someone call them back within a specific amount of time and move on to the next patient.

6. AVOID DEADLY PHRASES

Certain phrases only make angry patients angrier.

"I disagree..." versus "I understand, let's discuss the problem."

"Let's compromise..." versus "Let's find a solution by working together."

"It's our policy..." versus "This is why it is our policy."

"You have to"... versus "Here's something you may wish to try."

7. FOLLOW UP

The best way to turn an angry patient into an appreciative and loyal friend for the future is to DO WHAT YOU SAY YOU ARE GOING TO DO and follow up on it. In some cases, making a return call to ensure that the plan has worked out satisfactorily may be an excellent investment of time for both staff and patient satisfaction. It shows that you really do care.

8. TAKE A BREAK

When it is all over take a mental and physical time out as a way of dealing with "phone stress." If the call turned out well, congratulate yourself on a job well done, and share the experience with others.

CHAPTER 7

Guidelines for Patients: How to Use The Telephone More Effectively

When a patient selects his or her primary care physician (pediatrician, family practitioner, or internist), a patient-physician team is formed. If the patient is a child-parent combination, the whole family joins. As a team member, the patient has certain responsibilities. The more actively these responsibilities are taken, the more effective the telephone will work for the entire team.

1. Be Informed
2. Be Descriptive
3. Be Assertive
4. Be Understanding
5. Be Prepared

1. BE INFORMED
- Learn your doctor's phone system.
- Ask questions.
- Who answers the phone—nurse or non-nurse?
- Does your doctor work with nurse practitioners? What is their role?
- Are there specific call-in times?
- Can you speak to the doctor if you want to?
- If you want an appointment, and say so, do you get one?
- Under what circumstances might you use the hospital emergency room?
- One of the ways you can save time is to avoid peak telephone hours when calling in for routine appointments. Peak times should be reserved for acute and urgent problems requiring same-day appointments, peak hours include: early mornings, late afternoons, when children get home from school, and the day after a three-day weekend.

- Calls for routine appointments should be made in mid-morning or early afternoon. This smooths out telephone traffic so that you can be served more promptly. This consideration will be greatly appreciated by your physician and the office staff.

2. BE DESCRIPTIVE

- When you call your doctor's office, describe the problem objectively and to the point. Present an accurate history with the relevant details: "My daughter, Susan, is 6 years old and has had a loose chest cough and fever for the past 5 days. One Tylenol every 4 hours and lots of fluids are not working. Today, she has a temperature of 103 degrees, is much worse, and I would like to bring her in to see the doctor this morning." This is much more effective than "Susan isn't feeling well today and feels warm. I'm not sure what to do." The latter scenario will require more time and may not achieve what you really want.

3. BE ASSERTIVE

- If you are placed on "hold" before you get a chance to say anything, call back and object. This is unsafe because you might be reporting an emergency. Let the doctor or office supervisor know if you are dissatisfied.
- Feedback about the telephone system, both positive and negative, is important.

4. BE UNDERSTANDING

- Calls of an emergency nature will be given priority.
- If the appointment you are given conflicts with a personal commitment, it may be necessary for you to rearrange your schedule. This will allow the health center to better serve your needs. Your doctor's office will appreciate your flexibility in scheduling appointments.

5. BE PREPARED

- When you call, always have a pencil and pad next to your telephone for writing instructions.
- Take the temperature in advance of the call—you'll save time.
- Have a medicine chest well-stocked with the essential home treatment supplies.
- Keep frequently used telephone numbers near your telephone for quick reference.

6. THE WELL-STOCKED MEDICINE CHEST
- Medications (dose and indication to be prescribed by your physician).

Analgesics (for pain) and *Antipyretics* (for fever)
- acetaminophen (Tylenol, Tempra, Panadol—tablets, syrup, elixir)
- acety/salicyclic acid (aspirin). NEVER use aspirin for influenza or chicken pox because of possible link to Reyes' syndrome. If in doubt, use acetaminophen.
- Ibuprofen (for teenagers on advice of your physician)

Decongestants
- Sudafed (elixir—30 mg. per teaspoon; tablets—30 mg and 60 mg per tablet.)
- nosedrops (NeoSynephrine, Afrin)

Antihistamine
- Benadryl (elixir 5—12.5 mg per teaspoon, tablets—25 mg and 50 mg per tablet)

Emetic
- Syrup of Ipecac-to induce vomiting. (Give ONLY upon advice from physician or Poison Control Center never decide by yourself.)

Lotions and ointments
- *Nivea*
- *Calamine lotion (not Caladryl)*
- *Bacitracin or neosporine antibiotic ointment*
- *Vitamin A & D ointment, Vaseline*
- *Zinc oxide*

First aid and miscellaneous equipment
- Thermometer
- Assorted Bandaid sizes
- Ace bandages (2", 4" and 6" sizes)
- Kling gauze wrap (2" and 3" Sizes)
- Tape
- Gauze pads
- Splint
- Scissors and tweezers
- Calibrated measuring spoon

FREQUENTLY USED PHONE NUMBERS

- **EMERGENCY NUMBERS**

  Ambulance _____

  Police _____

  Fire Dept. _____

  Hospital _____

  Health Ctr. _____

  Other _____

- **PHYSICIANS**

  Pediatrician _____

  Internist _____

  Family Doctor _____

  OB/GYN _____

  Surgeon _____

  Dentist _____

  Other _____

  Other _____

- **IF YOU BELONG TO AN HMO**

  Pharmacy _____

  Urgent Care _____

  Claims Office _____

  Member Service _____

  Billing Office _____

  Other _____

  Other _____

CHAPTER 8

The Medical History

The most helpful part of the evaluation of any medical problem is the history, or narrative, of the illness. The physical examination usually confirms the history in establishing the proper diagnosis. The least important part of the evaluation is the use of laboratory tests. In the real world of a busy pediatric or family practice, the keys to a good history are relevance (selecting the most important questions that yield the greatest amount of useful information); the ability to judge the relationship the physician has with the patient and family as a means of assessing the validity and objectivity of the reported information; and finally, the art of being a good listener—for both facts and feelings. There is little time for a long, detailed discussion when there are several other patients *on hold,* impatiently waiting to present their problems. Decisions have to be made quickly and accurately. If there is an illness-related call from a new patient whose medical and social background is unknown, an appointment should be made immediately. The same is true for someone who is agitated or whose language is difficult to understand. All doctors have experienced, during their medical school training in history-taking, a case workup where a long time has been spent nervously taking the clinical history and performing the physical examination without gaining any real insight into the patient's problem. The precepting attending physician then walks in, puts the patient at ease within seconds, gently asks one or two probing questions (which the medical student somehow over-looked), and within minutes has the answer to the patient's problem. This is what is meant by relevance.

The medical history is an objective way of learning as much as possible about the patients' symptoms and the factors that may be influencing the problem, and it can be an effective means of assessing the needs of a patient in a telephone encounter. For telephone assistants, it may be helpful to review the components of a complete history as it is practiced by physicians when the patient is seen in the office. The same general approach is applicable over the telephone. The component parts of a medical history include the following:

- Chief complaint
- History of the present illness
- Review of systems
- Past, family, and social history

The chief complaint (cc) is defined as the reason for the patient's call and the description of the problem stated in the patient's or parent's own words. It is not a diagnosis.

For example, "my child has an ear infection" is not a chief complaint when the parent actually said "my child has an earache." The historian should note the chief complaint verbatim. Other examples of chief complaints might include "fever," "not feeling well," "failing in school," or "fussiness." It is vital for the person answering the telephone to appreciate the specific reason why a patient is calling by practicing the art of listening. The chief complaint is the portion of the history that is the introduction to the other parts.

The following examples illustrate how the history of the present illness (HPI) provides the background for the chief complaint, supplemented by a search for associated symptoms using a review of systems, and the past, family, and social components of the narrative.

REVIEW OF SYSTEMS

A review of systems is defined as a survey of all organ systems (head, eyes, ears, nose, throat, lungs, heart, abdomen, genitourinary, and neurological). The survey should be relevant to the present illness, such as questioning the mother of a child with a fever about the genitourinary complaints of burning on urination or frequency as a clue to the presence of a urinary tract infection. Parents frequently do not offer this information spontaneously if their focus is on another symptom. Probing a review of systems fits quite naturally into the body of the present illness when talking to parents. The nature of the complaint will determine how extensively and which systems should be surveyed. For example, extensive questioning about neurological symptoms is appropriate for a child with head trauma, but less relevant if the complaint is abdominal pain.

PAST, FAMILY, AND SOCIAL HISTORY

For the purpose of telephone medicine, the past history deals with any pertinent information about the child's past that relates to the present illness. Details about the child's birth, any previous serious illnesses, hospitalizations, or drug allergies that bear on the present illness or may influence therapy are to be included in the past history. For example, a child who has had a seizure is always questioned about any previous traumatic episode in which there may have been injury to the brain. It is important to know if a patient presenting with diarrhea has had a similar episode in the past that may have led to hospitalization for intravenous treatment of dehydration as a means of gauging the potential course of this illness. A child exposed to chickenpox will be managed quite differently if he or she is on chemotherapy for cancer or on steroid medication for kidney problems. This stresses the importance of always determining if there is any chronic underlying or coexisting disease. In the same way that a past history provides meaningful information, so too does a family and social history. A strong family history of diabetes, thyroid, or kidney disease may have a direct bearing on a child's illness. Social history includes sensitive information about family structure, school performance, and substance abuse. However, it is inappropriate for telephone assistants to obtain the details of this delicate and confidential history, which is reserved for the privacy of an office visit. On the other hand, the clue to the presence of a socially problematic situation is often picked up over the phone and should be relayed as such to the physician scheduled to see the patient.

In summary, one can view the parts of a history as components that should dovetail into a cohesive, logical picture of the patient's problem. The skills needed to accomplish this quickly and accurately over the telephone come with practice and experience.

As indicated above, the HPI is the patient's opportunity to detail the specifics that characterize the chief complaint. In an orderly fashion, the patient is encouraged to narrate the development, nature, and chronology of the symptoms as background to the chief complaint. For example:

CC: A 9-year-old complains of a stomachache.

HPI: The pain is dull and achy, started around the navel, and moved toward the right lower side of the abdomen. It began last night, steadily grew worse, and is now associated with fever of 102°F (rectal) and vomiting. The child has vomited twice in the past 2 hours, and is now refusing to eat or drink. There has been no diarrhea or urinary tract symptoms.

CC: The parent states that her 2-year-old has diarrhea.

HPI: For the past 2 days the patient has had eight watery bowel movements that do not contain blood or mucus. He is acting listless, has a temperature of 103°F, and has vomited once today. There has been no urine in the past 8 hours. Liquid nourishment is refused. The father had a similar illness 4 days ago and recovered without specific treatment.

CC: Fever of 102°F.

HPI: This 3-year-old girl has a slight runny nose but is otherwise alert and active. She is playful, and, although her appetite has fallen off a bit, she is drinking well. The cold has been present for the past 2 days and does not seem to be getting worse. She is not particularly fussy or lethargic.

The key to taking a history over the telephone is relevance and a quick, but complete, review of systems as a way of determining the nature of the problem and whether an appointment or home management advice is needed. Asking the right questions is discussed in Section II.

CHAPTER 9

Medico-Legal Issues in Telephone Medicine

Telephone medicine has become the newest medico-legal threat. As mentioned in Chapter 1, a Midwest jury recently found a medical group negligent in a case that was decided solely on the basis of advice given to parents by a registered nurse. The charge of malpractice and jury trial occurred 10 years following the incident. The parents alleged that the nurse should have insisted that their 2-year-old child be seen by a physician immediately, and that her telephone advice caused a delay in the diagnosis of the Hemophilus influenza meningitis that left her profoundly deaf and retarded. The child had been examined and diagnosed as having a viral illness by her pediatrician 36 hours prior to the critical telephone encounter when the parents called to report on her progress and requested advice. Expert witnesses for the defense testified that there was considerable evidence that the nurse did indeed offer an appointment which the parents declined, and proceeded to offer appropriate symptomatic home advice for fever and hydration management. The nurse was a member of a nurse counseling service organized and trained by her employers, a group of four highly regarded, board certified pediatricians. The parents, 10 years later, stated they recalled the specifics of the telephone encounter during which they reported to the nurse that their child was much worse, irritable, and listless. The main reason why the plaintiff's version was more believable to the jury was the actual telephone log of that day, which was retrieved from storage, photographically enlarged, and displayed boldly on the wall of the courtroom facing the jurors.

It was remarkable that the log still existed. It was also very damaging to the defense. Words such as fussy, listless, and temperature were recorded in such a way that they could have meant anything. The plaintiff's lawyers had a field day. The physician's examination notes in the medical record prior to the call were never called into question. The jury's decision rested primarily on the telephone encounter entry in the log book. In the end, they concluded that the nurse failed to follow established guidelines.

Much can be learned from this case study. A number of preventive measures can be taken that can improve the quality as well as reduce liability.

1. Time should be devoted to improving telephone systems and management, acknowledging that the vast majority of problems are caused by the system and not the staff.
2. Medically significant calls should be documented in the medical record.
3. We should write smarter, not longer.
4. Written decision guidelines and procedures are essential.
5. Training opportunities should be available for staff.
6. There should be clarity about who is responsible for what.
7. Risk management issues should be discussed with all staff
8. There should be a low threshold for appointments.
9. Supervision and consultation should always be available to staff.
10. Evaluation and review should be integrated into the system and documented.

A telephone encounter form is recommended as a means of regularly recording basic information in order to document the content of each medically important telephone encounter for future reference. Formats vary, ranging from a portable pocket-sized pad adapted for after-hours use to a detailed form with a pretaped backing suitable for entering each telephone encounter into the patient's medical record. A sample of the kind of information that might be recorded is presented in Table 6.

A sample telephone encounter form appears in Figures 4 and 5. At first glance, the forms may appear cumbersome, but as personnel become familiar with the format, recording of the relevant information during the conversation becomes second nature, with no loss of efficiency. For example, if a child is given an appointment because of an earache, only the identifying information and *earache* is written and the *appointment disposition* is checked. On the other hand, if a mother calls for advice in the management of an illness that requires home care instructions that include aspirin dosages, this should be *detailed in the advice section* succinctly and selectively. The encounter form can be ordered with a self-sticking adhesive back so that telephone encounters can be easily inserted into the patient's chart in chronological order as desired, or printed on both sides for maximum economy.

There are several reasons for written documentation of all medically important phone conversations and retaining them. Pertinent details of past conversations, as well as the date and name of the office personnel who received the call, can be quickly retrieved. This is invaluable if the patient subsequently presents a complaint, and past history must be separated from intervening events in an attempt to objectively evaluate the problem. Also, in a group practice, it is helpful for the physician on call to be able to

40

Table 6
INFORMATION THAT MIGHT BE RECORDED AS A RESULT
OF TELEPHONE ENCOUNTER

Identifying information
    Name
    Age
    History number
    Home phone
    Identity of caller
    1. Mother
    2. Father
    3. Other
Complaint or purpose of call
Outcome of call
    Appointment advised
    Call referred to (specify): _____
    Home management advice given:
    1. Independently
    2. Consulted with (specify): _____
    Patient told to return call: yes _____ no _____
Home management advice and treatment
    Description

Message for clinician to call patient back
    1. Nature of problem and urgency
    2. How soon call-back is expected

review details of prior telephone instructions when the patient's regular physician is away. Also, if follow-up information needs to be conveyed to a patient, or if instructions need to be changed or modified, it is helpful to have the patient's telephone number and details of the earlier call readily available. In some practices the records of all telephone encounters are kept in the patient's medical chart. The guidelines for which types of calls are to be recorded into the medical chart should be developed by the supervising physician. Finally, information about the number and type of telephone calls can be obtained easily for use by the physician(s) in discussions about staffing and telephone service, as modifications or expansion becomes necessary.

TELEPHONE ENCOUNTER

CALL RECEIVED BY _____ DATE _____ MORN ___ AFT ___ EVEN ___

NAME _____ AGE ___ CMP# _____ PHONE _____ CALLER: Mother ___
                                                                          Father ___
COMPLAINT _____ FU _____ Other ___
or
PURPOSE _____

OUTCOME CI ___ ADV ___ (to decide, did you consult with md ___ pnp ___ ha ___ cht ___)
  ADVICE   home care advice, sick child _____   t.c. requested _____
    IS   home care advice, well child _____   rx ___ rx refill _____
              lab result given   _____   obs. recall   _____
              school/other form info   _____   other _____
CALL REFERRED TO _____WE WILL CALL BACK _____

NAME _____ AGE ___ CMP# _____ PHONE _____ CALLER: Mother ___
                                                                          Father ___
COMPLAINT _____ FU _____ Other ___
or
PURPOSE _____

OUTCOME CI ___ ADV ___ (to decide, did you consult with md ___ pnp ___ ha ___ cht ___)
  ADVICE   home care advice, sick child _____   t.c. requested _____
    IS   home care advice, well child _____   rx ___ rx refill _____
              lab result given   _____   obs. recall   _____
              school/other form info   _____   other _____
CALL REFERRED TO _____WE WILL CALL BACK _____

NAME _____ AGE ___ CMP# _____ PHONE _____ CALLER: Mother ___
                                                                          Father ___
COMPLAINT _____ FU _____ Other ___
or
PURPOSE _____

OUTCOME CI ___ ADV ___ (to decide, did you consult with md ___ pnp ___ ha ___ cht ___)
  ADVICE   home care advice, sick child _____   t.c. requested _____
    IS   home care advice, well child _____   rx ___ rx refill _____
              lab result given   _____   obs. recall   _____
              school/other form info   _____   other _____
CALL REFERRED TO _____WE WILL CALL BACK _____

NAME _____ AGE ___ CMP# _____ PHONE _____ CALLER: Mother ___
                                                                          Father ___
COMPLAINT _____ FU _____ Other ___
or
PURPOSE _____

OUTCOME CI ___ ADV ___ (to decide, did you consult with md ___ pnp ___ ha ___ cht ___)
  ADVICE   home care advice, sick child _____   t.c. requested _____
    IS   home care advice, well child _____   rx ___ rx refill _____
              lab result given   _____   obs. recall   _____
              school/other form info   _____   other _____
CALL REFERRED TO _____WE WILL CALL BACK _____

Figure 4

Sample of telephone encounter form. There are four entries on each side separated by perforations (total of eight per sheet). Forms also come with pretaped backing for easy transfer to the medical record (total of four encounters per sheet). Abbreviations used (CI = come in; ADV = advised; pnp = pediatric nurse practitioner; ha = health assistant; cht = chart; t.c. = throat culture; rx = prescription; and obs. = observe)

HCHP: Braintree Telephone Encounter

Date: _____

Patient: _____
       FIRST   LAST

Provider: _____ Time: _____

Caller: _____
     (IF NOT PATIENT)

Phone #'s; NOW: _____ Until: _____

Unit # (or D.O.B.): _____

Phone #'s: THEN: _____ Until: _____

Urgency: ☐ - Immediately ☐ - w/in 1 hour ☐ - This Session

             ☐ - Call back not necessary ☐ -

Message (Not for input)

Message Taken by: _____

Diagnosis			(Below this line for Provider/Input Only)
	A117P	Viral Illness	
	A803X	Test Result Only	
	A128P	RX Refill Only	
Therapies			
	Y8333	Illness Mgmt.	
Referrals			
	42	Referral	Provider: _____

Figure 5

Figure 5. Note the urgency section for call backs indicating when return call is expected.

CHAPTER **10**

 # Objectives and Use of the Handbook

There are three major objectives of this telephone care manual: (1) to increase the telephone assistant's knowledge, and, therefore, the relevance of questions, decisions, and quality of advice when evaluating childhood illnesses presented by parents via the telephone; (2) to serve as a guide to a structured training program for individuals who will assume a telephone care responsibility; and (3) to stimulate the objective evaluation of the telephone assistant's knowledge of telephone care management by providing some basic audit tools. The manual speaks for a total telephone care system, but it is important to adapt the material to the content and philosophy unique to the individual practice setting and the socioeconomic characteristics of the population being served. There really should be no difference between a clinic and an office setting if the clinic is organized and supervised properly. Telephone care is not solely an exercise in triage, which means "sorting out." The telephone assistant must also be trained to exercise independent and informed judgment.

One of the most frequent questions parents ask their physician is, "When in the course of my child's illness should I see a doctor?" Unfortunately, there are no hard and fast rules. The safest response is that a child should be seen whenever parents are worried about how their child is acting in response to a given illness. However, decisions by parents about the appearance of their child during an illness are often made at home quite independently. At one end of the spectrum, a mother instinctively decides that her child is playful, not very ill, and that a call to the doctor is unnecessary. At the opposite end, a child appears so listless and irritable that medical attention is sought immediately. It is in between these two extremes that it may be unclear whether or not an appointment is really indicated. Decision-making in the gray zone, and sometimes even in the extremes, varies tremendously from parent to parent. An appropriate balance between the benefits versus the risks of home management for a given medical situation, and sound, informed judgment, are required for the best decision-making.

Regardless of how anyone feels about giving medical advice over the telephone, the fact is that it is done all the time in every office or clinic. It happens whenever patients call and the physician is out of the office, detained by an emergency, or tied up with other patients. Often, the person entrusted with the responsibility of responding to calls from patients is incompletely equipped for such an extremely important function. This may lead to errors in management, delays in getting appropriate medical attention, and also unnecessary office visits for problems that actually are better managed at home. Not all patients who are ill need to see a doctor, and it is physically impossible for all phone calls to be managed by the physician.

The telephone decision guidelines are directed towards helping parents decide when it is safe not to bring a child into the office for an appointment and what to do and look for while the child is being observed at home. They also contain information about when it is important to visit the doctor. The objective of this manual is to help promote a more informed decision-making process. The most common symptoms were selected on the basis of a study of the frequency distribution of approximately 2,5000 calls received over the course of 1 month in a pediatric department within a combined prepaid, fee-for-service multispecialty group practice. Each symptom in the manual has been divided into four interrelated subsections: a discussion of the general medical background information for a given medical problem; decision guidelines that include practical home management advice; (Section II); and an audit-evaluation approach adapted for office use; with relevant references selected for office personnel to stimulate additional reading. In a busy practice, it is not a realistic expectation that all relevant questions be used for every complaint. Time does not permit the luxury of a complete history; nor is one always needed. When a patient and his past history are well known, fewer questions will be necessary compared to a new patient. However, health professionals should know what questions are important in those situations where further history and evaluation of a problem are needed, and when time permits.

The Decision Guideline Key indicates the question to be asked in the left column and the corresponding suggested response on the right. Symbols are included which guide the timing of the apointment, i.e., STAT (immediately); the same session, as soon as possible; the same session but with no urgency; the same day (afternoon is appropriate if the morning session is either inconvenient or already booked; or a future appointment.

Stat	☆☆	Same Day	●
Same Session ASAP	☆	Appointment (24–72 hrs.)	□
Same Session	○	Appointment (4 days or more)	■
High priority items are shaded			

It is emphasized that these suggested responses are guides and can easily be modified according to individual clinician preferences.

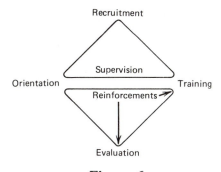

Figure 6

Key factors in developing a telephone care system.

The second major objective of the manual is to serve as a guide to a structured training program. The training objective can take many different forms, and emphasizes the importance of the key factors seen in Figure 6. Perhaps the most important factor is the type of person selected for the position. The manual should be studied thoroughly by each telephone assistant as part of training and orientation. The decision guidelines can be used as the basis for role playing sessions in which the supervising physician or nurse assumes the role of parent. This can be performed as a one-on-one exercise or in a group discussion format between junior and senior health assistants. A suggested training schedule is presented in The Four-Step Approach (see pg. 202).

A structured training approach in telephone care is applicable to several types of health professionals. A number of studies have indicated that physicians, nurses, nurse practitioners, health associates, as well as pediatric and family practice house officers could all benefit from additional training in telephone medicine.

The third objective of the manual addresses the concept of evaluation of the telephone care system and personnel. For the most successful program, it is important that the telephone responsibility be integrated into the fiber of the medical practice. It is a dynamic role and should be periodically reassessed and modified, striving for the highest quality performance. The collection of data on number and time of peak calls is helpful in this regard, as is the careful analysis of patient complaints, which may lead to improvements in the system as a result of problem solving. The performance of the telephone assistant must also be monitored. A basic audit form has been designed to assess whether key questions are asked during role playing sessions between, for example, a physician and nurse, or while listening in to a real conversation between a parent and the assistant. In this way the supervising health professional can engage the telephone assistant in meaningful educational dialogue. This process should take place with all new personnel and should be repeated periodically with the more senior staff so that the supervisor can readily evaluate the capabilities and judgment exercised by telephone assistants. The atmosphere initially might be somewhat inhibited, but with gentle encouragement, personnel quickly relax, particularly when the constructive and educational objective of the audit exercise is emphasized—rather than it being just a *quiz*. Importantly, these sessions also enable the physician to impart his individualistic approach to both the evaluation and management of specific illnesses, and stimulate the telephone assistant by providing continuing medical education, a sense of teamwork, and bonding between support staff and clinicians.

REFERENCES

Katz HP, Pozen J, Mushlin AJ: Quality assessment of a telephone care system utilizing non-physician personnel. *Am J Public Health* 1978; 68:31–38.

> *This paper presents (1) a descriptive analysis of 2,500 telephone calls to an office practice, (2) a quality assurance study of the performance of non-physician, nonnursing personnel trained in triage and to offer home management advice via telephone, and (3) a description of the training process for these pediatric health assistants and the telephone care system in which they functioned.*

Reece RM, Robertson LS: The telephone answering service—A survey of use by general practitioners and pediatricians in Massachusetts. *Clin Pediatr* 1972; 11:40–43.

> *A summary of an after-hours answering service confirmed that much more medical advice is offered by untrained personnel than is either delegated or perceived by physicians.*

Section II

Symptoms, Decision Guidelines, and Home Management Advice

CHAPTER **11**

Fever

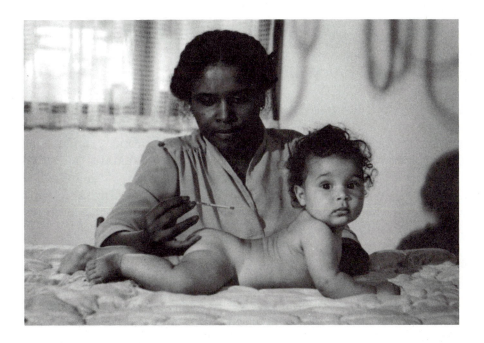

One hundred twenty-two years ago, routine temperature taking was first advocated as a means of following the course of childhood illness. As useful as this has been, few symptoms have generated more anxiety than fever, as any parent who has watched the mercury column shoot to 105°F will agree. Unfortunately, much confusion and misunderstanding has surrounded the meaning and management of this symptom. It is very important for telephone care providers to understand fever's significance, and also the guidelines for its management.

WHAT IS TEMPERATURE?

As a result of the study of temperature patterns in 25,000 individuals, the following facts are known:

1. Children have less precise temperature regulation and higher normal temperatures than adults. Infants have higher basal temperatures than do older children.

2. The normal range of body temperature is from 97°F–100.4°F, rectally, and between 96.8°F–99.3°F, orally.
3. The maximum temperature occurs between 5:00 and 7:00 P.M.
4. Because the temperature can be 100.4°F (rectally) in an active, normal child, fever is defined as an abnormal increase in body temperature beyond this level. The questions frequently asked by parents include:

IS HIGH FEVER HARMFUL?

Contrary to popular belief, fever is rarely dangerous or harmful to the brain, even at levels of 104°F lasting for several days. In fact, fever is a sign that the body's defense mechanism is working properly, and it actually helps fight the infection. In the 1- to 5-year age group, fever may precipitate a convulsion; however, evidence suggests that it is the rate of rise rather than the actual height of fever that sets off the seizure. A febrile seizure occurs very early in the course of the illness and often precedes the awareness that fever is present.

WHAT DOES FEVER MEAN?

Fever is a normal response to infection. *The degree of fever is not a true indicator of the severity of illness.* A temperature of 103°F is really no different from one of 101°F. A benign illness with minimal symptoms, such as the common cold, may be associated with a temperature of 105°F, while an extremely serious infection may have little or no fever. *It is important to identify the type of infection that is causing the fever.* The nature of the symptoms, the clinical findings, and appropriate tests reveal this. Because fever above 102°F can by itself cause symptoms such as listlessness, it is advisable to lower the fever in order to define symptoms more objectively and to help the child feel better. One should not feel as if something has to be done. If the child does not appear ill, no treatment of the fever is necessary.

MANAGEMENT OF FEVER

This information refers primarily to the older child. While a child is being observed at home, or after the nature of illness has been defined by the physician, the appropriate dose of antifever medication should be used for maximum benefit. A child may be kept comfortable and side effects of the medication minimized by prescribing the correct dose of either aspirin or acetaminophen-containing drugs, as seen in the following chart.

Table 7
FEVER MANAGEMENT MEDICATION CHART

Drug	Strength	Less Than 6 Mos	6 Mos–1 Yr	1–2 Yrs	2–3 Yrs	3–5 Yrs	Over 6 Yrs
Baby aspirin	1¼ grains or 80 mg/tablet	*	*	One	Two	Three or four	*
Adult aspirin	5 grains or 325 mg per tablet	*	*	*	*	*	One
or							
Tempra or Tylenol drops	80 mg per 0.8 cc	½ Dropper 0.4	1 Dropper 0.8	1 Dropper 0.8	2 Droppers 1.6 cc	*	*
Tempra or Tylenol elixir	120 mg per tsp (5 cc)	*	*	½ tsp	1 tsp	1½ tsp	2 tsp
Chewable Tylenol tablets	80 mg per tablet	*	*	One-half to one	One to one and one-half	Two	*
Adult Tylenol tablets	325 mg per tablet	*	*	*	*	*	One

*Not recommended.** Evidence indicates a *possible* association between aspirin and Reyes syndrome. Until further information becomes available, the academy of pediatrics advises against the use of aspirin for proved or suspected cases of chickenpox and influenza.

- Give medicine every 4 hrs until fever is under 101°F or child is comfortable.
- Do not give more than the recommended dose (use as prescribed by your doctor).
- Do not sponge with cold water or alcohol.
- Increase the intake of fluids (popsicles, juice, flat sodas, jello water).
- Do not leave unused medication within reach of child, and always replace cap immediately.
- Acetaminophen preparations contain different concentrations. Always read the label carefully for recommended dosage.
- Dosage of acetaminophen is 5 to 7.5 mg per pound of body wt (maximum 600 mg at any one time).

Following is a chart offering decision guidelines. Questions in the left column correspond to suggested responses in the right columns. High priority items are shaded.

FEVER

	QUESTION	TO SEE DOCTOR IF . . .	
1.	Age of child.	Under age of 6 mos. regardless of anything else (greater than 100⁴ F rectally).	○
2.	How long has fever been present and what is the actual temperature?	Fever present more than 48 hours without explanation, or any fever over 103°F.	●
3.	How is your child acting?	Child appears unusually ill, irritable or lethargic.	☆☆
4.	Has your child ever convulsed?	Yes.	○
5.	What is your child's usual state of health?	There is any chronic disorder, such as diabetes, cystic fibrosis, asthma, seizures, etc.	
6.	Are there any other symptoms? (See below for review of Symptoms.)	The review of systems indicates a serious source of infection.	
	Head (CNS)	Headache is out of proportion to fever. Stiff neck.	☆☆
	Ear, nose, throat (ENT)	There is a cough, sneezing, sore throat, earache, or swollen glands.	●
	Respiratory	There is rapid breathing or difficult swallowing present. Cough	☆☆
	Gastrointestinal (GI)	There is vomiting, diarrhea, or abdominal pain.	○
	Urinary (GU)	There is burning or frequency. What is fluid intake? Amount and type?	●
	Skin	There is a rash (i.e., petechial).	☆☆
7.	Is there anyone at home with similar symptoms?		

Stat	☆☆	**Same Day**	●
Same Session ASAP	☆	**Appointment (24–72 hrs.)**	□
Same Session	○	**Appointment (4 days or more)**	■

High Priority Items are shaded

54

QUESTION	TO SEE DOCTOR IF . . .	
8. What is the dose of aspirin or acetaminophen (Tylenol, Tempra, Liquiprin) that has been given at home?	Child has received an excessive dose.	

Stat	☆☆	Same Day	●
Same Session ASAP	☆	Appointment (24–72 hrs.)	☐
Same Session	O	Appointment (4 days or more)	■

High Priority Items are shaded

ADVICE

Child should be seen if there is any doubt as to the seriousness of the illness.

The illness may be treated by phone advice under the following conditions:

1. If the child is not acting particularly ill, fussy, or lethargic.
2. If there are associated respiratory or gastrointestinal symptoms that are mild and the above review of systems is essentially negative.
3. If there is mild illness in other family members with similar symptoms.
4. If the parent feels comfortable with the home advice disposition.

The parent should always be instructed to call back if the symptoms are worsening or changing significantly.

Aspirin or acetaminophen may be prescribed as follows:

Aspirin

1. **No aspirin for chickenpox or influenza-like illness. If any doubt, use acetominophen.**
2. A safe rule is to administer two baby aspirin for children age 2–3 yrs; and three baby aspirin for age 3–5 yrs.
3. After the age of 5, four baby aspirin or one adult aspirin may be given every 4 hrs.
4. *Always replace cap and keep out of reach when not in use.*

Acetaminophen (Tylenol, Tempra, and Liquiprin are brand names) 5–7.5 mg per pound of body wt with a maximum of 600 mg at any one time.

1. Drops—80 mg per 0.8 cc (Liquiprin is 60 mg/1.25 ml)
2. Elixir and Syrup—120 mg/tsp (5 cc)

55

Elixir and Syrup	*Drops (preferred for infants)*
Under 1 yr—½ tsp every 4 hrs 1–3 yrs—½–1 tsp every 4 hrs 3–6 yrs—1½ tsp every 4 hrs	0.4–0.8 cc/4 hrs

Sponging Instructions

Sponging is only an adjunct recommended for the relief of symptoms when the fever is over 103°F. Relief is only temporary. The principle is to promote heat loss via evaporation, similar to the cool feeling experienced when leaving a swimming pool.

1. Use plain water at room temperature. *Do not* use ice or alcohol since these might cause shivering, which raises body temperature.
2. *Do not* immerse the body in water or cover with wash cloths. This impedes evaporation.
3. Rub a wet cloth or sponge briskly over the arms, legs, and trunk, and then let the water evaporate from the surface of the skin.
4. Stop sponging if shivering occurs.
5. Sponge for only 15–20 minutes. By then the medication has begun to work.

Fever is a healthy sign that the body is responding to infection and is not harmful. It actually helps fight infection. Treatment objectives are to (1) make the child more comfortable, and (2) reduce the possibility of a fever convulsion in children between 1 and 5 years old. Treating fever does not treat the illness.

CHAPTER **12**

Colds and Earache

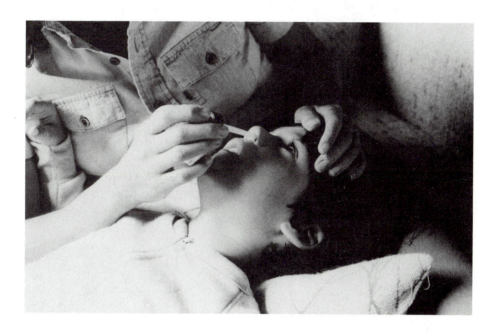

THE COMMON COLD

Sir William Osler, the famous Hopkins physician at the turn of the century once said, "There is only one way to treat a cold—and that is with contempt." It is a distressing experience for most parents to watch their children suffer through a bad cold. Understanding and sympathy by medical professionals are essential ingredients of treatment. Parents are understandably frustrated. Children miss school, working parents must take off from work, baby-sitting arrangements are complicated, elective surgery must be postponed, and vacation plans are delayed. When one cold follows another in a large family, someone is always ill. Everyone is on edge and wants a cure. However, overtreating the cold with unnecessary medication does not help, and may cause harm.

Science has not yet discovered the cure for the common cold. The prevention of colds by vitamin C has not been documented. Although there is no drug cure, cold symptoms can be relieved by simple medication. Which medicine to use remains controversial. Antihistamine pills and decongestants may reduce nasal congestion but do not shorten the duration of the cold. The same effect can be achieved by the judicious use of gentle nose drops without making the child drowsy (which antihistamines may do). Other drugstore cold remedies often contain a mixture of three or four different ingredients, some of which are of very questionable value. Importantly, the risk of serious side effects is increased when multiple ingredients are administered.

What about antibiotics for a cold? A cold is caused by a virus, and since antibiotics do not work against most viral infections, antibiotics will *not* influence the common cold. There is also no evidence that antibiotics will reduce the complications of colds for most children. There is one more reason why over-medicating should be discouraged, and that is to avoid creating in the child the attitude that the ills of life should be treated by pills. The more we learn about drugs, the more caution we feel is necessary in their usage. Life is not, as all too many people feel, a drug deficiency.

When a child has a cold the objectives of management are twofold: to make our patient comfortable, and to alert the family to signs that there may be a complication of the cold, such as an ear infection, sinus infection, pneumonia, or bronchitis.

EARACHE

There are basically three types of ear infections, all of which make their presence known by causing ear pain. They are

1. *Exudative otitis media:* bacterial infection of the middle ear.
2. *Serous otitis media:* fluid in the middle ear often associated with bacterial infection, but also associated with other causes.
3. *Otitis externa:* external ear infection, swimmer's ear.

The following lists present the salient features of the first two types. It is important to stress that combinations of either two or all three types can be present in one patient. The symptom common to all types is pain, and all patients need to be seen for an examination in the office.

Exudative Otitis Media	*Serous Otitis Media*
Marked ear pain and/or throbbing that usually occurs 2 to 3 days af-	Fleeting ear pain, discomfort, "popping," or feeling of stuffiness.

ter an uncomplicated cold. Less commonly, the onset is abrupt and unexpected.

Commonly associated with irritability and fever. Often there is ear-tugging by infants and young children unable to verbalize their complaints.

Decreased hearing or disturbed balance, on occasion.

Discharge of pus or blood from the ear (signifies rupture of eardrum). This sometimes causes an associated external canal infection.

Increased incidence in allergic patients.

Decreased hearing and to a lesser extent, balance, are common.

May be associated with discharge of sticky fluid as eardrum ruptures from pressure buildup.

Treatment of otitis media is aimed at minimizing pain and discomfort, treating the infection with specific antibiotic therapy, and allowing aeration and drainage from the middle ear to return to normal function with reopening of the eustachian tube (the tubelike structure that connects the middle ear to the area behind the nose). If antibiotic treatment is prescribed, it must be continued for the full 10-day course of therapy. Maximal compliance with the treatment plan is essential and should be reinforced by instructions whenever possible.

Otitis Externa

Otitis externa, or ''swimmer's ear,'' is an infection of the skin that lines the ear's outer canal, commonly associated with swimming in pools during the summer. It can also result when the eardrum ruptures during an episode of otitis media with discharge of pus and bacteria into the canal. The presence of moisture in the ear canal softens the skin and provides a favorable environment for infection. Pain is occasionally severe, and there may be fever. A hallmark of this condition is marked pain when the outer ear is moved or touched, a situation not observed in the more common middle ear infection (otitis media). Most cases of otitis externa will respond to antibiotic–cortisone ear drops used four times daily for 7 to 10 days. In cases where significant swelling or discharge is present, it sometimes is necessary to insert a cotton wick, saturated with Burow's solution, into the ear canal to help reduce the swelling. Pain is relieved by aspirin and gentle heat applied over the outer ear by means of a heating pad or hot water bag. It is important that instructions be followed carefully since this usually mild disease may worsen and cause severe pain if treatment is incomplete. In cases where improvement is not seen within 36 to 48 hours, or if symptoms are worse, the child should be seen for further evaluation.

Following is a chart offering decision guidelines. Questions in the left column correspond to suggested responses in the right columns. High priority items are shaded.

COLDS AND EARACHE

QUESTION	TO SEE DOCTOR IF . . .	
1. Age of child.	Per physician's preference.	
2. How long has cold been present?	Longer than 4 days and getting worse.	○
3. Are there any associated symptoms: Earache Sore throat Other	See below. See sore throat section. Child is acting particularly ill. Fever is greater than 102°F for more than 48 hrs. If productive or persistent cough or chest pain is present. Severe headache or stiff neck. Sinus headache or congestion is suspected.	 ○ ● ○ ☆☆ ●
4. Does your child have any other serious medical disorder?	Child has diabetes, asthma, nephrosis, or heart disease.	☆
5. Is fever present?	Fever is greater than 102°F and present for longer than 48 hrs.	●
6. Is earache present (or if earache is present complaint)?	All patients with earaches should be given appointments, to be seen as soon as possible. Few questions need to be asked. The only considerations are: (a) Whether the appointment should be immediate (come right in). (b) Advice to make the patient comfortable until the appointment. The following situations warrant an (a) Parents and child up all night.	● ☆

Stat	☆☆	**Same Day**		●
Same Session ASAP	☆	**Appointment (24–72 hrs.)**		□
Same Session	○	**Appointment (4 days or more)**		■

High priority items are shaded

QUESTION	TO SEE DOCTOR IF . . .	
6. (Continued)	(b) Distraught parents.	
	(c) Severe, unrelenting pain. (Make sure aspirin is given before the trip to the office.)	○

Stat		★★	**Same Day**	●
Same Session ASAP		★	**Appointment (24–72 hrs.)**	□
Same Session		○	**Appointment (4 days or more)**	■

High priority items are shaded

ADVICE

- If an antihistamine is advised (e.g. Chlor-Trimeton), indicate that it may make child drowsy. If this occurs, discontinue the drug.

- If an oral decongestant (e.g. Sudafed) is used instead of nose drops and antihistamines, indicate that this may cause a mood change or hyperactivity. If this occurs, discontinue the drug.

- Children may return to school and should no longer be considered infectious when there has been no fever for 24 hrs and symptoms have either been gone or minimal for the past 24 hrs.

also

- Encourage a liberal fluid intake—water, juice, chicken broth, especially when cough and fever are present.

- Rest.

- **Saline nose drops for young infants (This can be purchased in drugstores). Administer 2 drops in each nostril 3 times each day for two days.**

or

- **Neosynephrine nose drops (⅛% for young children 1–6 yrs). Do not use for more than 3 days or more than three times a day.**

- **Chlor-Trimeton syrup (2 mg/5 ml) given as 1 tsp 3 times a day (2–8 yrs).**

or

- **Sudafed Syrup (30 mg/5 ml) given as ½ tsp three times a day (1–2 yrs) and 1 tsp three times a day (2–12 yrs).**

- **Sudafed Tablets (60 mg/tablet) given as 1 tablet three times a day (over 12 yrs).**

To Make the Patient with an Earache More Comfortable While Waiting for an Appointment:

1. *Aspirin*—A safe rule is to administer two baby aspirin for children age 2–3 yrs; three baby aspirin for age 3–5 yrs. After the age of 5, four baby aspirin or one adult aspirin may be given every 4 hrs.

   Always replace cap and keep out of reach when not in use.

   If influenza or chicken pox is suspected, no aspirin should be used.

   or

   Acetaminophen (Tylenol and Tempra)

   Elixir and Syrup—120 mg/tsp

   Elixir and Syrup

1–3 yrs	½–1 tsp every 4 hrs
3–6 yrs	1½ tsp every 4 hrs

2. Gentle heat applied to the outer ear by means of a heating pad, hot water bottle, or warm wash cloth.

3. Auralgan ear drops if they are available in the home (do not use if discharge is noted). Three drops of warmed Auralgan in the affected ear with a cotton pledget to seal ear canal as a single dose.

CHAPTER **13**

 # Sore Throat

Infection of the tonsils and throat (pharynx) is the major, but not only cause of a sore throat. The medical terms that describe the infection are tonsillitis, pharyngitis, and pharyngotonsillitis. Most infections involve both the tonsils and pharynx, therefore, these two structures can be viewed as a combined anatomical unit (Fig. 7).

Infections of the throat may be caused by both viruses and bacteria. The vast majority of infections are viral. The symptoms subside spontaneously and are not improved by antibiotic treatment. Unfortunately, it is not possible to know whether the infection is viral or bacterial by inspecting the throat. For this reason, a throat culture has become a useful tool in helping to decide between the two possibilities. Results of the throat culture usually are available within 24 hours.

The most common bacterial cause of sore throats is the "strep" germ, an abbreviated term for the bacteria called *Streptococcus*. For practical purposes, the major question to answer about the cause of a throat infection is, "Is it a 'strep' or not?" Other bacterial causes besides strep do not have to be considered unless there are special reasons. This is important to know because a number of other bacteria normally live in the human throat but do not cause infection or symptoms. The primary purpose of a throat culture is to identify the specific kind of strep germ (there are many different types) that causes infection, which, if not treated properly, can lead to complications, such as rheumatic fever (arthritis and heart problems) and nephritis (bleeding into the kidney and urine). Treatment of strep throat consists of antibiotics, usually penicillin, if the child is not allergic to this drug.

Response to treatment of a strep throat usually is rapid and successful. However, it is not uncommon for the strep to survive treatment, and for symptoms to recur. Parents should not become overly frustrated if this happens to their child. In this situation, a cause for the persistence of a strep germ can usually be determined and the problem solved by the physician. Detailed discussion between the parent and doctor may focus on subjects such as, why some children may not absorb oral antibiotics well enough from their stomach, and therefore require injections rather than oral medication; whether the child is actually taking the medicine (compliance); spreading of the strep germ within a family (ping-pong effect); when it may be appropriate for other family members to be cultured; the carrier state (strep in the throat but no symptoms); and lastly, the role of tonsillectomy in the management of recurrent streptococcal throat infections. Each of these subjects must be individualized and requires close communication between patients and their physician in order to avoid misinterpretation about the reason and significance of recurrent or repeated throat infections. Fortunately, the vast majority of children do not present this problem. Whenever they do, the telephone assistant's role is to recognize the recurrent nature of the problem and refer the case to the family's regular physician.

Following is a chart offering decision guidelines. Questions in the left column correspond to suggested responses in the right columns. High priority items are shaded.

TELEPHONE DECISION GUIDELINES
SORE THROAT

QUESTION	TO SEE DOCTOR IF . . .	
1. Age of child.	Under age 4 yrs.	
2. How long has sore throat been present? Is throat sore just in morning versus continuous?	Present more than 12 hrs and continuous. All children with significant sore throats should have a throat culture. This can be done either in the office, or . . . see Advice.	●
3. Is fever present?	Yes.	●
4. Are glands in the neck swollen and/or tender?	Yes.	●
5. Is there a cold or cough?	Yes.	●
6. Is there a rash, headache, or stomachache?	Yes.	●
7. Has child had many sore throats or streptococcal infections before?	Yes.	●
8. Is there a stiff neck?	Yes, see immediately.	☆☆
9. Is child acting particularly ill?	Yes.	☆
10. Is the child seen for any other chronic illness?	Yes (diabetes, asthma, nephrosis, congenital heart disease, etc.)	☆

Stat	☆☆	**Same Day**	●
Same Session ASAP	☆	**Appointment (24–72 hrs.)**	□
Same Session	○	**Appointment (4 days or more)**	■

High priority items are shaded

*Not with chickenpox or influenza

HOME THROAT CULTURE OPTION

The purpose of the home throat culture approach is to involve parents more directly in the diagnosis of their children's streptococcal throat infections by doing the throat culture at home, in lieu of an office visit. Some parents wish to participate more closely in the diagnostic process, particularly when families are large, have young children (between the ages of 4 and 10), or have children who are more susceptible to recurrent streptococcal sore throats. There are many potential advantages to this approach, and some disadvantages (Table 8).

It is important that a patient's physician agree with the concept of a home culture approach. Some favor this strongly, others feel the opposite. A physician must supervise the training of parents and provide the necessary follow-up. It should be stressed to parents that a child is never placed on an antibiotic without first being examined. Interested parents are shown a diagram of the throat with written instructions (Fig. 7) and then are instructed by a member of the office staff in the technique of swabbing. Indications for culture, namely uncomplicated sore throat of greater than 12 hours duration with or without fever, are discussed and parents are given a supply of Culturette tubes to be taken home and used as needed. If the culture is positive, the patient is called in, examined, and treated as deemed appropriate by the physician. Patients are told they will receive no call if the culture is negative, and that they may assume the cause of the throat infection is most probably viral and will get better

Table 8
POTENTIAL ADVANTAGES AND DISADVANTAGES OF A HOME THROAT CULTURE PROGRAM

Advantages
1. Promotes informed parent participation in children's health care.
2. Promotes increased awareness of the importance of cultures.
3. Promotes education regarding specific antibiotic therapy.
4. Decreases unnecessary office visits.
5. Prompt and accurate diagnosis.
6. Reduction in cost of medical care.
7. Decreases contagion.
8. Decreases child's anxiety by less exposure to physician.

Disadvantages
1. Taking throat cultures improperly and missing the strep.
2. Taking too few cultures.
3. Taking too many cultures, thereby increasing laboratory burden and cost.
4. Taking cultures when a visit is indicated by the presence of other symptoms.
5. Creating friction between parent and child.

spontaneously. However, if they received no call and their child becomes worse, the child should be examined. A study (Katz & Clancy, 1974) was done which confirmed the validity and safety of this approach. Furthermore, it was postulated that the home culture approach might also provide benefits in terms of early detection of illness, efficiency of health delivery, decreased costs, more appropriate utilization of health services, and increased convenience for patients who voluntarily choose to participate.

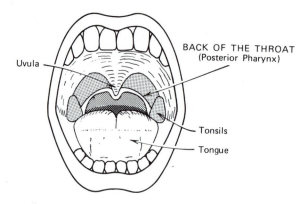

**Throat Culture Instructions
for Home Culture Program**

1. **Why Take a Throat Culture?**
    Since it is impossible to determine, merely by inspecting the throat, whether a throat infection has been caused by a virus or by the **Streptococcus** germ (strep throat), a throat culture is needed. There are also signs that the doctor looks for on examination, to determine whether an individual should be placed on an antibiotic before the culture results are known. If those signs are not present, there are very good reasons to wait 24 to 48 hours until the results of the throat culture are reported. This will eliminate unnecessary use of antibiotics.

2. **Symptoms and Major Indications for Doing a Culture**
    a. Sore throat with or without fever.
    b. Upper respiratory symptoms after being exposed to a strep infection.

3. **Obtaining a Throat Culture:**
    a. On the white paper portion of the Culturette, please write your child's name, phone number, and history number.
    b. Remove the cotton swab from its container.
    c. Swab several times over both tonsils and back of throat (see diagram).
    d. Return swab to its container, and replace its white cap.
    e. Crush the capsule around the liquid container, and bring the specimen directly to our laboratory as soon as possible.

4. If the culture is positive within 24 to 48 hours, **we will call you** and write a prescription for antibiotics which must be continued for 10 full days. If you do not hear from us, you can assume the throat culture was negative. In this case, the inflamed throat was most probably caused by a virus and should clear up within a few days. If you are concerned by a persistent illness, please call us for evaluation.

Figure 7

Sample of printed instructions to be given to those parents trained to perform home throat cultures. The shaded areas indicate the areas of the throat to swab with the Culturette.

CHAPTER **14**

Cough and Wheezing

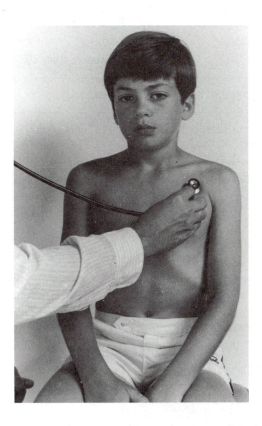

There are many causes of a cough, which can be separated into two basic groups: those in which the cough originates in the upper airway (above the lungs) versus a cough that is associated with disease in the lower airway (lungs). Examples of upper airway factors include the following:

- Local irritation secondary to environmental factors, such as cigarette smoke.
- Dryness from lack of humidity in the home.
- Postnasal irritation of the throat caused, for example, by hay fever or the nasal discharge of a cold dripping into the throat.
- Sore throat caused either by the common cold or the *Streptococcus*.
- Croup.

TELEPHONE DECISION GUIDELINES
COUGH AND WHEEZING

	QUESTION	TO SEE DOCTOR IF . . .	
1.	Child's name, age, and duration of cough.	If less than 3 yrs, has a temperature, or cough been present for 2–3 days without improvement.	○
2.	Are there any associated symptoms? • Chest pain • Fever	Yes. Greater than 102°F.	☆
3.	Does child appear very ill?	Yes.	☆
4.	Has child been seen previously for this illness?	Yes, and getting worse.	○
5.	Is child wheezing or asthmatic?	Yes.	☆
6.	Is cough • Dry or loose • Productive of mucus • Waking child from sleep • Mild and associated with cold • Croupy, barking	Loose and productive. Yes. Refer to section on colds. Refer to section on croup.	○ ○
7.	Is child breathing differently from normal, such as: • Faster • Harder or more shallow • Grunting or noisy Chest caving in and out	Yes.	☆
8.	Does child have a serious chronic medical problem?	Yes.	○
9.	Are there members of the family ill with similar symptoms		
10.	Is child being given any medications now?		

Stat	☆☆	**Same Day**	●
Same Session ASAP	☆	**Appointment (24–72 hrs.)**	□
Same Session	○	**Appointment (4 days or more)**	■

High priority items are shaded

- A foreign body, such as a peanut, that is aspirated into the lungs.
- A fish bone caught in the tonsil (which also may be associated with spitting blood).
- Laryngitis.

Coughs in this group of disorders are not appreciably relieved by patent cough medicines. Except for the nonspecific effect of the syrup and alcohols on the irritated throat, cough syrups do not treat the root cause of the cough. The soothing effect on the throat also can be achieved by a mixture of tea, lemon, and honey, which is considerably less expensive than cough medication, and eliminates the use of alcohol. The cessation of smoking by parents, the use of antihistamines for nasal allergy, and a steamy bathroom for croup are specific treatments for individual underlying causes in the upper airway-induced cough.

Cough caused by disease of the lower airway, such as pneumonia, asthma, or bronchitis, is a protective mechanism which clears the lungs by bringing up mucus. Expectorants loosen up the mucus. One of the best expectorants is drinking liquids, such as water, juice, or soup. Asthma is an allergic disorder in which there are recurrent episodes of wheezing sometimes associated with upper respiratory infections or pneumonia. Pneumonia means infection has developed within the lung tissue and air sacs. Wheezing associated with asthma can be described as a squeaky musical sound which is made when a child exhales or breathes air out of the lungs. Breathing is often strained and respirations are rapid. Wheezing and cough are caused by the combination of tightness, spasm, and mucus in the bronchial tubes. All children who are wheezing should be seen by the physician for specific treatment. Parents quickly learn how to evaluate the response to previously prescribed medication and know when their child should be seen because home treatment is not progressing satisfactorily.

The accompanying chart of Decision Guidelines indicates questions in the left column and corresponding suggested responses in the right column. High priority items are shaded.

ADVICE

- If cough is mild and associated with a cold, or if child is having throat irritation because of nasal mucus dripping into the throat, advise parent to give a mixture of warm tea, honey, and lemon.

- If there is a great deal of associated nasal congestion or sneezing, decongestant (Sudafed) or antihistamine (Chlor-Trimeton) may be advised, and occasionally an expectorant (Robitussin), if congestion involves the chest.

- Under some conditions a cough suppressant may be indicated, particularly if the cough is exhausting the child and family for lack of sleep. Cough suppressants should be advised by or in consultation with the physician.

- Fever management should be advised per previous section.

Drug	Under 1 Yr	Age of Child		
		1–5 Yrs	6–12 Yrs	Over 12 Yrs
Decongestant				
Sudafed (30 mg/tsp)	Not recommended	½ Tsp. 3 times daily	1 tsp. 3 times daily	2 tsp or 1 tab 3 times daily
Antihistamine				
Chlor-Trimeton syrup (2 mg/tsp)	Not recommended unless specified by M.D.	½ tsp 3 times daily	1 tsp 3 times daily	1 tsp or 1 tab 3 times daily
Expectorant				
Robitussin	Not recommended	½ tsp 3 or 4 times daily	1 tsp 3 or 4 times daily	1 or 2 tsp 3 or 4 times daily

CHAPTER **15**

Croup

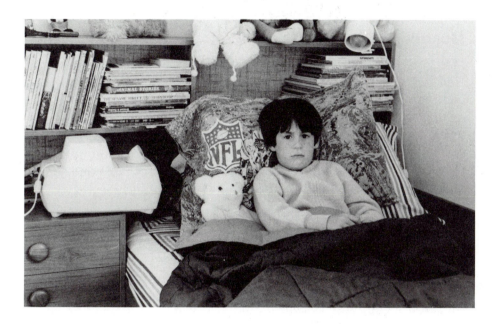

Croup is a disorder characterized by a cough that sounds like a barking seal or a foghorn. It is also accompanied by noisy respirations (stridor), primarily during inhalation (breathing in), and varying degrees of difficult breathing. The stridor is caused by breathing in through a narrowed windpipe at the level of the larynx (voicebox) and trachea (windpipe). In contrast, low airway obstruction (narrowing) results in wheezing or difficulty exhaling (breathing out), as in asthma. There are 4 basic types of croup: (1) viral inflammation of the larynx and trachea; (2) inflammation of the epiglottis (structure that covers the trachea when swallowing food); (3) spasmodic (midnight) croup; and (3) foreign body croup.

CROUP CAUSED BY A VIRUS

This is the most common form and occurs most often in children between 6 months and 4 years of age. It may be caused by the same viruses that cause the "common cold." After several days of cold symptoms, the child develops a barky cough, noisy breathing, and in bad cases, may strain to breathe. Fever is usually mild and the child does not appear ill. When the lower airway is also involved, wheezing may accompany the croup. More severe airway narrowing leads to retractions of the chest wall while breathing, because of difficulty in getting enough air into the lungs past the narrow voicebox.

Management

Mist inhalation is very effective in reducing the swelling of the upper airway. Humidifying the bedroom with a vaporizer or sitting in a steamy bathroom with the child cuddled in the parent's arms are the best treatment. Vomiting may give dramatic relief. Antibiotics are not indicated unless there is secondary bacterial infection, as in an ear infection. Patent cold medicines do not help and may actually make croup worse by excessive drying of secretions. If there is high fever or rapid and strained breathing, the child should be seen in the office at once.

INFLAMMATION OF THE EPIGLOTTIS (EPIGLOTTITIS)

This form is caused by a bacterial infection and generally affects older children between the ages of 3 and 7 years. It is rapidly progressive and dangerous. The onset is usually abrupt with fever, strained breathing, pain on swallowing, drooling, and severe sore throat. The voice may sound muffled, and the child appears quite ill.

Management

The child should be given an immediate appointment. Epiglottitis is an emergency situation.

SPASMODIC (MIDNIGHT) CROUP

Spasmodic croup can affect any age group and recurrences are quite common. Onset is sudden, usually at night or nap time. There is a barky cough, noisy respirations, and little else. This form rarely progresses to airway obstruction. The symptoms usually abate during the day and return at night for several days. Sitting in a steamy bathroom for 15 minutes is most helpful. The child should be cuddled in the parent's arms and both should try to be as calm as possible. Reading a story often helps relax the child.

Following is a chart offering decision guidelines. Questions in the left column correspond to suggested responses in the right column. High priority items are shaded.

TELEPHONE DECISION GUIDELINES
CROUP

QUESTION	TO SEE DOCTOR IF . . .	
1. Name and age of child?	Less than 1 yr.	○
2. How long has the croup been present?	Longer than 3 days.	○
3. Is fever present?	Greater than 102°F.	○
4. Is child making a loud noise when he/she takes a breath?	Yes.	☆
5. Is child's chest caving in as he/she breathes?	Yes.	☆
6. Is child breathing rapidly?	Yes.	☆
7. Does child look ill or pale?	Yes (immediate visit).	☆☆
8. Does child look frightened?	Yes (immediate visit).	☆☆
9. Is child drooling or having difficulty swallowing?	Yes (immediate visit).	☆☆
10. Do lips or skin look bluish?	Yes (an emergency).	☆☆
11. Has the child choked on something small that could have stuck in his/her throat?	Yes (immediate visit).	☆☆
12. Has child been exposed to a similar illness?		
13. Is child playful and drinking fluids well?		
14. Are there any other associated symptoms?		
15. Does child have any other serious medical problems?	Yes.	●
16. Are you giving child any medication?		

Stat	☆☆	**Same Day**	●
Same Session ASAP	☆	**Appointment (24–72 hrs.)**	☐
Same Session	○	**Appointment (4 days or more)**	■
High priority items are shaded			

ADVICE

If child is playful, alert, and drinking fluids well, and if the croup is mild with no respiratory difficulty, then home management is appropriate provided the child will be observed closely.

- Steam up the bathroom by running hot water from the shower. Close the door and sit in the thick steam with your child held on your lap for about 10 min. Do this three or four times during the day.
- Use a cool mist vaporizer in the child's bedroom. No medication needs to be added to the water. Run vaporizer continuously.
- It is very important to relieve your child's anxiety by calm reassurance.
- Parent to call back immediately if any of symptoms (questions 5–10) develop.

Parents should check the child frequently. The barking cough will persist. However, as strained breathing develops or worsens, then an evaluation in the office is advised (either first or repeat visit). Parent should sleep in room with child for closer observation.

CHAPTER **16**

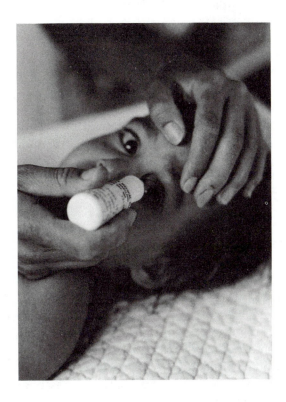 **Eye Infection and Inflammation**

Inflammation of the lining over the white of the eye (conjunctiva) may be bacterial, viral, allergic, or traumatic (mechanical or chemical injury) in origin.

BACTERIAL CONJUNCTIVITIS

Purulent (pus) discharge and crusting of the eyelids may occur with intense redness of the eye in the bacterial type. The infection is contagious, and may last for several weeks if untreated. An appointment is required for all cases, to confirm the diagnosis and to rule out other associated infections, like otitis media. The most effective treatment consists of antibiotic eye drops. If the symptoms become worse while using the eye drops, an allergic reaction to the drops or the need to change to a more effective eye preparation should be considered. To prevent spread of infection, separate cloths or wet cotton balls should be used for cleansing the eyes. The child is considered noncontagious when the redness and signs of illness have been gone for 24 hours.

VIRAL CONJUNCTIVITIS

Viral conjunctivitis also may cause redness of the conjunctiva and either a watery or purulent discharge. There is no specific treatment for viral conjunctivitis, but secondary bacterial infections are treated with antibiotic eye drops. Since viral conjunctivitis is a diagnosis of exclusion, most patients should be given appointments for an examination.

ALLERGIC CONJUNCTIVITIS

In spring and fall many patients with allergies develop eye symptoms. Itching, swelling, and a watery discharge are common in children with associated hayfever or asthma. The conjunctiva becomes red, which is increased by rubbing. Cool compresses afford some relief, together with mild vasoconstricting eye drops and oral antihistamines. Since it may be difficult to distinguish allergy from infection, patients are best seen. An exception can be made when the condition has been previously diagnosed, the pattern is similar, and the medications have been successful in prior seasons.

NONSPECIFIC REDNESS

External irritants, such as smoke, smog, fumes, swimming pool chlorine, ocean water, or factors such as inadequate rest or eyestrain, may produce conjunctival redness. A complete eye examination should be performed if the symptoms are associated with a change in vision, or if there is doubt about the cause. Elimination of the offending agent is the treatment.

CONJUNCTIVITIS OF THE NEWBORN

Any inflammation of the conjunctiva of the newborn is considered to be in this category. The inflammation may be due to the chemical irritant, silver nitrate, which is placed into the eyes to prevent gonococcal infection, or to other infections, bacterial or viral, acquired from an infected birth canal during delivery. Any inflammation of the conjunctiva of the newborn should be seen by the physician for proper diagnosis and treatment. Excessive tearing and recurrent inflammation in the first few months of life may indicate a blocked tear duct, a common pediatric problem that is usually self-limiting.

STY

A sty is an infection at the base of the eyelash, usually caused by the *Staphylococcus* organism. It can be treated with warm compresses and a topical antibiotic ointment applied four times a day. If the eyelid is very red or swollen, the child should be seen in the office.

Following is a chart offering decision guidelines. Questions in the left column correspond to suggested responses in the right column. High priority items are shaded.

EYE INFECTION AND INFLAMMATION

QUESTION	TO SEE DOCTOR IF . . .	
1. Name and age of child?		
2. How long has the eye symptom been present?	Longer than 24 hrs.	○
3. Is the white of the eye very red?	Yes.	○
4. Is there pain?	Yes.	○
5. Is there a thick discharge or crust?	Yes.	○
6. Is the eye swollen?	Yes.	○
7. Was the eye injured either by an object or chemical substance?	To be seen immediately if yes.	☆☆
8. Do the eyes itch?	Yes.	○
9. Has he/she had this before?		
10. Are you using any medication now?		
11. Are there associated symptoms: • Wheezing? • Fever? • Earache? • Redness of the skin around the eye?	Yes. Yes. Yes. If yes—appointment as soon as possible.	○ ○ ○ ☆
12. Does the child appear ill?	Yes.	☆
13. Does child also have a cold?		
14. Does the child have a sty or pimple at the base of the eyelash?	Eyelid is very red, tender, or swollen.	○

Stat	☆☆	Same Day	●
Same Session ASAP	☆	Appointment (24–72 hrs.)	□
Same Session	○	Appointment (4 days or more)	■

High priority items are shaded

ADVICE

If this is a recurrent allergic problem and the family has used medication before, they can be instructed to use it again and report back in 24 hrs. Be sure the episode is similar, and has been diagnosed and treated as allergic by a physician in the past. If there is doubt, the child should be seen.

If the child has a mild cold and the eye has been only faintly red for less than 24 hrs., warm washcloth compresses to soothe the eye can be tried for 24 hrs. If symptoms increase or persist, the child should be seen. (In many instances, the infection is a mild viral one and the eye infection clears by itself.) If there is doubt, the child should be seen.

If the sty is a small pimple, advise warm compresses with a warm washcloth (which has been placed under the hot water tap). It should be rewarmed each time it cools, for a total soak time of 10 min, four times a day. A prescription for a topical antibiotic ointment can be obtained from the physician.

If there has been injury by a chemical substance, rinse the eye thoroughly for 10 minutes with water immediately. Hold the eyelids open under running water from a faucet or hose. See a doctor at once.

CHAPTER **17**

Diarrhea and Vomiting

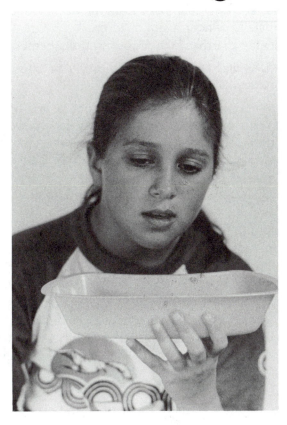

Diarrhea is defined as an abnormal increase in either the number or water content of bowel movements. There are many causes of diarrhea. If the diarrhea is chronic (lasting longer than 1 week), an appointment is needed for an evaluation in the office. More commonly, the complaint is one of acute symptoms of recent onset. The cause of acute diarrhea is most often a viral infection of the intestinal tract (gastroenteritis). In young infants, diarrhea can also develop because of food intolerance (milk protein allergy: lactose or milk sugar sensitivity). In addition, loose stools are frequently associated with upper respiratory illness, especially ear infections.

Diarrhea caused by infection with intestinal viruses usually disappears within several days. Marked diarrhea with mucus or blood in the stool, and diarrhea associated with high fever and acute illness should be given an appointment, since a bacterial organism may be identified. After the initial infection is over, secondary milk sugar intolerance can prolong the recovery rate. Therapy of diarrhea is aimed at preventing dehydration by providing adequate fluid intake, and resting the bowel by avoiding solid foods. Medicines, such as paregoric, Lomotil, and Kaopectate are ineffective and potentially dangerous in children.

For uncomplicated diarrhea, the following management is suggested:

1. All solid food, as well as milk and milk products, should be withheld for approximately 24 to 48 hours.

2. During this period, fluid intake should be liberal and consist of water, weak sweet tea, non-red Jell-o water (1 package per quart of water) or, for the older child, soft drinks, such as flat gingerale, cola, or 7-Up. A special electrolyte solution called Pedialyte can be prescribed for infants. Fluids should be offered every 2 to 3 hours. Pretzels, soda crackers, or dry toast, if desired, may be given to older children.

3. For infants and younger children, on the second or third day, half-strength skim milk or half-strength formula may be started with gradually increasing small amounts of bland solid food, such as applesauce, lamb, boiled chicken, rice cereal, and boiled rice.

4. On the third day, full-strength milk or formula and a regular diet can be resumed provided the diarrhea has responded well (a decrease in number and in volume of stools). If diarrhea persists, a trial of Isomil or ProSobee can be prescribed to eliminate lactose (milk sugar) from the diet.

5. Medications, such as Kaopectate, paregoric, or Lomotil, have no place in the routine treatment of diarrhea in children. They do not alter the course of the illness, and can be quite harmful since they may mask the amount of fluid loss into the bowel and cause serious side effects.

VOMITING

1. If vomiting is present, all solid food and liquid should be withheld for a short time until the child feels like drinking.

2. *Do not force* fluids if the child is nauseated: more will come back up than stays down.

3. Offer sips (by teaspoon) of cracked ice, water, coke syrup, flat gingerale, or cola.
4. If the child can keep down sips taken every 15 minutes, he/she can then be encouraged to take gradually increased amounts of clear liquids.
5. Maintain the child on clear liquids as outlined above for 24 to 48 hours. If desired, pretzels, soda crackers, or dry toast can be tried.
6. If vomiting is severe, or associated with abdominal pain, marked diarrhea, or is not responding to the above, a visit to the physician is indicated.

Following is a chart offering decision guidelines. Questions in the left column correspond to suggested responses in the right column. High priority items are shaded.

TELEPHONE DECISION GUIDELINES
DIARRHEA

QUESTION	SEE DOCTOR IF . . .	
1. Age of child.		
2. How long has diarrhea been present? Describe the kind of bowel movement.	Present more than 48 hrs.	●
3. How many diarrheal stools?	There have been more than 5–6 watery stools in large quantity within a 12 hr period in an infant.	○
4. Is there vomiting and abdominal pain also?	There is vomiting with right-sided pain.	☆☆
5. Is there blood in the stool?	Present.	☆
6. Is there much mucus in the stool? Does it look like pus?	Present.	○
7. Does child look unusually ill?	Yes.	☆☆
8. What is the usual state of child's health?	A significant chronic disease is present (such as diabetes).	○
9. Does the child appear dehydrated? Is mouth moist when last urinated?	*Dehydration* is suspected. See signs.	☆
10. Are there other symptoms: Fever? Breathing fast and hard? Jack-knifing knees to chest with severe cramps? Earache?	Over 103°F. Yes. Yes. Yes.	○ ☆ ☆ ○
11. Has child been exposed to a similar illness in family or friends?		
12. Has child been on a clear liquid diet?	Diarrhea not responding after 24 hrs on clear liquid diet.	

Stat	☆☆	**Same Day**	●
Same Session ASAP	☆	**Appointment (24–72 hrs.)**	□
Same Session	○	**Appointment (4 days or more)**	■

High priority items are shaded

88

ADVICE

If child is alert, active, and does not appear unusually ill, and if diarrhea is mild and infrequent (less than six stools in past 12 hrs without blood or mucus), then feeding advice and home management are appropriate.

Review of Diet

1. Clear liquids—Jell-o, weak sweet tea, flat sodas for 24 hrs or until diarrhea subsides. Offer liquids every 2 hrs. Pedialyte can be used for infants.

2. As diarrhea subsides, on second to third days, can progress, in infants, to BRAT diet (banana, dry rice cereal mixed with water, applesauce, and dry toast).

3. If child is under the age of 1 yr, diluted Isomil (formula containing no milk sugar) can be started after clear liquids ($\frac{1}{4}$ strength on first day, $\frac{1}{2}$ strength on second day, and then full strength). Continue full strength for 5 days. Can then resume normal formula or milk. Yogurt and cheese can be used earlier since they do not contain lactose.

4. If a diaper rash appears, use thick coat of vaseline to protect skin.

See fever management section if fever is present. Also see vomiting advice section if vomiting is present.

Signs of Dehydration

Listlessness
Dry tongue and inner cheek
Tears absent when crying
Sunken eyeballs
No urine in last 8–10 hrs

VOMITING

	QUESTION	TO SEE DOCTOR IF . . .	
1.	Age of child.		
2.	How long has vomiting been present?	More than 24 hrs in child on clear liquid diet with no improvement.	○
3.	How many times?	More than three times in the past 6 hrs.	○
4.	Does child appear unusually ill?	Yes.	☆
5.	Are other symptoms associated with the vomiting?	Any of the responses to the following questions (5 a-i) is yes.	
	a. Any severe headache or stiff neck?	See immediately.	☆☆
	b. Abdominal pain in right side?	See immediately.	☆
	c. Pain or burning on urination?		○
	d. Excessive irritability, listlessness, or mental confusion?	See immediately.	☆☆
	e. Earache, cold, sore throat?		●
	f. Severe diarrhea?		○
	g. Any blood in vomitus?	See immediately.	☆
	h. Breathing hard and/or fast?	See immediately.	☆
	i. Any exposure to a poisonous substance?	See immediately.	☆☆
6.	Fever?	Yes.	●
7.	What is usual state of health?	There is any chronic disorder, such as diabetes or asthma.	○
8.	Is anyone else in the family ill with similar symptoms?		
9.	Does he/she appear dehydrated: Is mouth moist? When last urinated?	Dehydration is suspected. See signs.	☆

Stat	☆☆	**Same Day**	●
Same Session ASAP	☆	**Appointment (24–72 hrs.)**	□
Same Session	○	**Appointment (4 days or more)**	■

High priority items are shaded

ADVICE

If home management is deemed appropriate, the following instructions should be followed:

Nothing to be given by mouth for 1 hr. Then, if child is younger than 18 mos, offer Pedialyte, weak sweet tea (barely color the water and sweeten to taste), or Jell-o water (5 cups of water to a package—don't use red color) for 24–48 hrs.

If older than 18 mos, offer ice chips, coke syrup, or sips of water (1–2 tsps for the first hr. If there is no further vomiting, offer flat soda, weak sweetened tea, Kool Aid, Jell-o water, crushed popsicles, or Gatorade).

Child should take an amount of clear liquids equal to or greater than the usual milk and fluid intake in a 24 hr period. Approximately 4–8 oz should be offered every 2-6 hrs for children over 1 yr.

If vomiting has ceased (none in past 12 hrs), child may proceed to toast, saltine crackers, and clear broth on the second day, and then gradually back to a normal diet.

Babies can be started on the BRAT diet (see diarrhea section).

Signs of Dehydration

Listlessness
Dry tongue and inner cheek
Tears absent when crying
Sunken eyeballs
No urine in last 8–10 hrs

CHAPTER **18**

 # Abdominal Pain

In ranking the frequency of middle-of-the-night calls from frightened parents, abdominal pain places high on the list, preceded only by high fever, earaches, and asthma. When children say their stomach hurts, parents immediately think of the appendix. Although this possibility always exists, it is uncommon. A thorough history, however, should always be taken, which focuses on whether a surgical problem may be present. There are countless other causes of abdominal pain in children, so it is important to consider the diagnostic possibilities, particularly as they relate to the child's age.

YOUNG CHILDREN (LESS THAN 2 YEARS OLD)

It is best for all young children with the complaint of abdominal pain to be examined, chiefly because they are unable to verbalize their symptoms. Abdominal pain in young children can be caused by stomach virus infections, food allergy, urinary tract infections, pneumonia, sickle cell disease, and not uncommonly, constipation. The probability of a surgical problem, such as intestinal obstruction, is increased when the parent reports that the knees are jackknifed, or drawn up onto the chest, or if the child appears pale and sweaty. Frequently, when the parent reports that the infant appears to have a stomachache, something else may be present, such as an ear infection. This is another reason why young children should be given an appointment rather than home advice.

OLDER CHILDREN (OVER 2 YEARS OLD)

The diagnostic possibilities in older children are best divided into those of either chronic or acute/short duration. If abdominal pain has persisted for months (chronic), then a future appointment is necessary. At this time, a detailed history and examination will be done to determine the cause, which can range from less common serious gastrointestinal disorders, like inflammatory bowel disease (Crohn's disease) and ulcers, to one of the most common causes of pain, namely, anxiety and tension (functional or psychogenic).

The most common cause of acute nonlocalized abdominal pain is an intestinal viral infection, or gastroenteritis. The location of the pain in the description is very important, since *any pain localized to the right lower side should be considered to be acute appendicitis until proved otherwise.* The typical history (and many cases are not typical) for appendicitis starts when the child loses his/her appetite, and at about the same time stomach pain appears. The pain usually appears around the belly button, then travels to the right lower side. Low-grade fever, nausea, and vomiting are accompanying symptoms. It is important to be aware that some cases of appendicitis are caused by and often follow an acute gastroenteritis. Other causes of abdominal pain in older children include hepatitis (inflammation of the liver), a twisted ovary in girls, a blow to the abdomen in a sports contest or accident, and pneumonia. In adolescents, venereal disease (gonorrhea) should be suspected.

In most instances of abdominal pain, home advice should not take the place of an examination. Once the diagnosis of a nonsurgical problem has been established by the physician, follow-up care can be augmented by sound telephone management focusing on the significance of changes in the child's condition and relief of symptoms, for example, as in gastroenteritis and fever management.

Following is a chart offering decision guidelines. Questions in the left column correspond to suggested responses in the right column. High priority items are shaded.

TELEPHONE DECISION GUIDELINES
ABDOMINAL PAIN

QUESTION	TO SEE DOCTOR IF . . .	
1. Age of child.	Infant is under 3 yrs of age or, if pain is accompanied by fusiness, vomiting, pallor, sweating, or if child appears ill.	☆
2. How long has pain been present?	Over 3 days duration.	○
3. How severe is the pain?	Severe, regardless of duration.	☆
4. Where is pain located?	Located on right side of the abdomen.	☆
5. Is it constant or intermittent?	Constant.	○
6. Is it getting better or worse?	Worsening.	○
7. Was there any tauma to the abdomen?	Yes.	☆
8. Are there any associated symptoms? Fever? Vomiting? Diarrhea? Difficulty breathing? Severe cough or chest smptoms?	Over 103°F or if fever is present longer than 24 hrs. See fever guidelines. Present. See diarrhea guidelines. Present. Present.	☆ ○ ○ ☆ ○
9. Are any family members ill with similar abdominal symptoms or with associated vomiting or diarrhea?		
10. Is child acting particularly ill or lethargic?	Yes.	☆
11. Has child been seen in the past for this problem?	Complaint is chronic, schedule a future appointment.	☐

Stat	☆☆	**Same Day**	●
Same Session ASAP	☆	**Appointment (24–72 hrs.)**	☐
Same Session	○	**Appointment (4 days or more)**	■

High priority items are shaded

QUESTION	TO SEE DOCTOR IF . . .	
12. What is usual state of health?	Any chronic condition is present.	
13. Have you been treating the child with any medications? Specify.		

Stat	☆☆	**Same Day**	●
Same Session ASAP	☆	**Appointment (24–72 hrs.)**	☐
Same Session	○	**Appointment (4 days or more)**	■

ADVICE

If the infant is under 2 mos and has symptoms of colic, an appointment with the doctor is important. Once the diagnosis has been established, subsequent phone calls are best referred to the physician because parents may become extremely distraught and need direct access to the doctor, who knows the patient best.

If symptoms of gastroenteritis are present and the pain is crampy, intermittent, and not severe or worsening, the child over 3 yrs can be observed at home and put on a clear liquid diet, with instructions to call back if the pain increases or localizes to the right side.

If the pain is intermittent and crampy and there has been exposure to a similar illness at home, which includes either vomiting or diarrhea, or both, then the child can be observed at home. A clear liquid diet should be prescribed for 24 hrs. If hungry, dry toast or saltine crackers can be tried. Parent should call back if child is worse or symptoms change.

CHAPTER **19**

Rashes

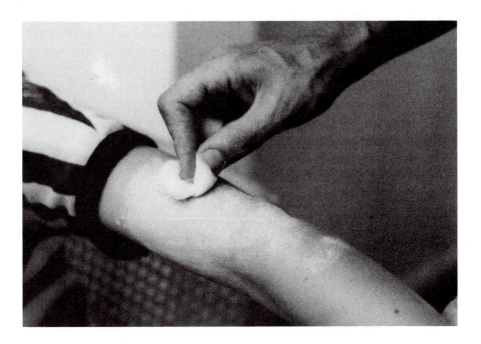

GENERAL INFORMATION

In most instances, rashes should not be diagnosed over the telephone. One look is worth a thousand words. It is simply easier, quicker, and much more accurate to diagnose a rash after a proper examination. There are, however, some notable exceptions. Chickenpox, for example, is an illness most physicians would prefer to keep out of their office because of the contagion aspect. Some skin conditions, such as eczema and diaper rash, may have been previously diagnosed, and the parent calls to request a refill of medication because her supply has run out. A reliable parent can assume some of the responsibility for diagnosis, as when a sibling has been in to see the doctor with a plantar wart, and sometime later another sibling develops the same kind of lesion. The main role for telephone advice in the case of rashes is clearly not diagnosis, but the dissemination of *patient education information* regarding

- Incubation period and duration of contagion
- Possible complications, such as secondary infection
- Treatment for relief of symptoms
- Follow-up expectations and instructions

There are countless skin disorders which, collectively, are one of the most common reasons why parents call their physician. For the telephone training purpose of providing general background information, the following rashes have been selected for discussion: warts, impetigo, poison ivy, eczema, diaper rash, petechiae, chickenpox, scarlatina, and drug rashes, all of which seem to generate the majority of phone encounters for rashes.

SPECIFIC INFORMATION

Warts

Warts are caused by a viral infection of the skin. Unfortunately, warts are often misunderstood and cause considerable emotional reactions on the part of patients. Warts are not a threat to a patient's health, and most of the time they will disappear without treatment. This may require several years. During this interval, the patient may acquire additional warts by self-inoculation of the virus from existing warts and also may be a contagious source of virus to other susceptible individuals. Treatment of warts should be appropriate to the age of the patient and to the size and location of the wart. Due to the discomfort of treatment and the young patient's difficulty with full cooperation, patients under 6 years of age should not be treated unless there are special circumstances, such as pain, bleeding, or when the wart is located on the face or close to the fingernail. Plantar warts are located on the bottom of the foot and should be removed because they are almost always quite painful. The very young child, those with a potential for poor cosmetic results, and warts that are complicated or widespread, should be referred to a dermatologist. These kinds of referrals should be rare. Reassurance to parents about the benign nature of warts, and that the long-term cosmetic results are best if the wart is permitted to go away spontaneously, usually convinces families to take a conservative approach.

When prescribing home methods of treatment, such as 40% salicyclic acid plaster or Duofilm (salicylic acid 17%-lactic acid 17% in flexible collodion), one should be specific about the method of application. Always discuss the size of the area to be treated, frequency of application, duration of treatment, and possible complications. (*Caution:* Avoid applying to normal skin.) The latter includes irritant dermatitis and infection. Follow-up appointment should be after an interval of several weeks to months.

The possibility of bacterial infection should not be overlooked. Any break in the skin, whether by rupture of a blister or fissure following use of wart medication, serves as a source of entry for bacteria. Good skin hygiene and the use of topical antibiotics, when appropriate, should be emphasized.

Impetigo

What Is It?/Where Does It Come From?

Impetigo is a common skin condition that occurs in many children and adults. It is an infection of the skin. Impetigo usually starts when there is a break in the skin's surface from a mosquito bite, scratch, or irritation of the nostril from a runny nose. Bacteria are then introduced, often by scratching. The most common bacteria are the *Streptococcus* and/or the *Staphylococcus*. A child scratches or rubs a lesion, the bacteria get on the fingers, which then spread the infection to other areas of the skin or to someone else. Bacteria can be cultured from the lesions, although routine cultures are not indicated in most situations because of the expense and ease of diagnosis visually.

How to Recognize It?

Although impetigo is relatively common, there are still many people who are unfamiliar with its appearance. The lesions usually begin as small red bumps but soon enlarge, become moist in appearance, and then develop yellowish crusts or scabs on a red base. When impetigo is caused by the *Staphylococcus*, the lesions generally appear as large, flat blisters filled with a milky fluid. These blisters can rupture, leaving raw areas of skin. This form is often seen in infants, but can appear in older children and adults as well. Impetigo is most prevalent during the summer months.

Is It Contagious?

Impetigo is contagious. Contaminated washcloths and clothing should be washed with either Lysol or Clorox. Children should be kept out of school or day-care until antibiotic treatment has been given for 36 to 48 hours.

Treatment

The most successful treatment for impetigo is an oral antibiotic. In those instances when there are only one or two very small lesions, topical treatment can be tried, washing with an antibacterial soap, like Dial, and applying Bacitracin Ointment, a local antibiotic ointment sold in pharmacies without a prescription. Patients may start topical therapy (four times a day for 1 week) when there is question of an early case, but if new lesions appear, or if the initial lesion enlarges, the child should be seen in the office and be considered for treatment with oral antibiotic therapy. The most common locations for impetigo are just below the nostrils, the chin, and on the extremities. Lesions can vary in size from approximately ($\frac{1}{4}$ inch in diameter to several inches across; and even the small lesions require treatment.

Potential But Uncommon Complications

It might appear that treatment is overly aggressive for a relatively mild skin disorder; however, the reasons for this are twofold. First, impetigo does not respond well to local treatment, and may spread to involve large areas of skin and underlying tissues. Secondly, glomerulonephritis, a specific type of kidney disorder characterized by bloody urine, may follow skin infections caused by certain strains of the *Streptococcus* bacteria. The same group A, beta-hemolytic strep that causes sore throats is the organism that causes impetigo. Fortunately, rheumatic fever has never been shown to complicate a case of impetigo. It is hoped that by prompt therapy, the possibility of nephritis can be prevented.

Poison Ivy

Poison ivy is a form of a contact dermatitis, which means that a substance has touched the skin and produced a rash—usually red, with tiny blisters—which is very itchy. The rashes of poison ivy, oak, and sumac are indistinguishable. These plants are easily recognized and bloom in profusion during the summer and fall. Children should be taught to identify poison ivy, by far the most common problem. If a child has been in contact with poison ivy, immediate thorough cleansing with a soap and water wash can lessen the dermatitis. Application of lotions, such as calamine, dry the skin and help relieve the discomfort. Benadryl, an antihistamine, can be prescribed for further management if the itching is troublesome. Rarely, cortisone medication (prednisone) is necessary for treatment of the rash and swelling. If the rash covers a large portion of the body, if it seems to be infected, if the eyes are swollen, or if there is extreme discomfort, the child should be seen.

Eczema

Eczema is a specific type of inflammation of the skin that occurs in children who have a genetic tendency toward allergy. The skin in eczema is red, swollen, itchy, often weeping with crusts and scales. The creases of the elbow and behind the knee are frequently involved. There is a close association between eczema and other forms of allergy, like hayfever and asthma. Children with eczema (sometimes called atopic dermatitis) have very sensitive skin that reacts more to other stimuli, like dryness and certain types of fabric. In the majority of children, the eczema either disappears or markedly improves by 5 years of age. Because of scratching, eczema frequently becomes secondarily infected. Any patient with a rash suspicious of eczema should be seen for treatment and a full discussion by the physician to promote a better understanding of this chronic disorder and its implications.

Diaper Rash

There are several causes of diaper rash. The majority of rashes in the diaper area are caused by the wetness and irritation of moist diapers rubbing against the skin. Treatment consists of air-drying the skin (a process speeded up by means of a hair dryer with a blower), changing diapers frequently, and applying a protective barrier, like Desitin or Vaseline. A diaper rash may become secondarily infected with bacteria or yeast. The most common secondary infection is with the yeast Candida, the same fungus that causes oral thrush and vaginitis. Whenever a diaper rash is reported to get worse or to look infected, the child should be given a same-day appointment.

Petechiae

Petechiae is a term that refers to a skin lesion, which is caused by bleeding into the skin. In contrast to a bruise, a petechia is a tiny pinpoint red dot. In most red rashes, if they are blanched (place each thumb on opposite sides of the skin lesion, press, and spread apart) the redness disappears. A petechia remains—it will not blanch. Petechiae may appear suddenly in crops or clusters on any part of the body. Any child with petechiae should be seen right away, because in some instances, this signifies the presence of a serious bloodstream infection. There are a number of less serious causes for petechiae, but an evaluation in the office is needed for specific diagnosis.

Chickenpox

There are more calls for chickenpox than most other rashes. As mentioned above, it is best to avoid an office visit for children with chickenpox, if appropriate. However, the child should be seen if:

- There is doubt about the diagnosis.
- The child appears very ill.

- The parent is anxious.
- There is a question of a complication, such as ear or eye infection, pneumonia, brain involvement, or secondary bacterial infection of one of the skin lesions.

The characteristics of chickenpox are the following:

- Multiple small blisters (vesicles) on a red base, often preceded by red raised bumps (papules).
- Pox, which at the outset are mainly located on the chest, back, and stomach.
- Breaking out that occurs in clusters, so that some clusters contain fresh lesions whereas others are older with black crusts already forming.
- An incubation period of between 11 and 21 days.

Nonspecific symptoms of fever, listlessness, or decreased appetite can precede the rash by 1 to 2 days. The rash begins suddenly with crops of raised red lesions (papules) that quickly form clear blisters (vesicles) on a red base. Contents of the blister become cloudy and then rupture, becoming scabbed or crusted over. Usually crops continue to erupt for about 3 to 4 days. When the entire rash becomes scabbed over, the child is no longer contagious. The rash also may involve mucous membranes (mouth, genitals), where shallow ulcers form. The severity of the disease varies from a few lesions with little toxicity to a widespread rash with high temperatures (102–105°F). The illness varies in duration between 5 and 14 days, the average being approximately 7 days.

Treatment is directed at making the child comfortable by reducing itching, pain, and fever. The risk of secondary infection as a result of scratching can be minimized by keeping the nails short. Secondary bacterial infection is treated with oral antibiotics. Symptoms are managed by the liberal use of tub soaks with oatmeal or bath oils, using acetaminophen for fever and antihistamines for mild sedation and the relief of itching.

Scarlatina

Scarlatina or scarlet fever refers to a "strep" throat plus a rash that is actually caused by an allergic reaction to the "strep" germ. It does not have the serious implications that existed in the preantibiotic era. It is really no different from strep tonsillitis, aside from the rash. The rash is very characteristic: tiny, raised, small bumps that are very red, and when gently rubbed, feel rough like sandpaper. The skin looks like a sunburn with goose bumps, and often peels (desquamates) in about 7 to 10 days.

Children with this kind of rash need a same-day appointment. Treatment with antibiotics is highly effective and there is no need for the anxiety that was present in preantibiotic days.

Drug Rashes

When a child who is on a drug develops a rash, it is important to rule out allergy to the medication. This is more likely to be the case if true hives are present. In the case of ampicillin or amoxicillin, between 5 and 10% of children develop a nonallergic nonspecific rash which is flat, pink, and not itchy. It usually lasts 3 to 4 days and requires no treatment. In most instances, an office visit should be given to document the nature of the rash for future reference, or the call should be referred to the physician to make the final decision. Advice should be given to discontinue the medication until the patient is seen or speaks to the doctor.

Following is a chart offering decision guidelines. Questions in the left column correspond to suggested responses in the right column. High priority items are shaded.

RASHES

QUESTION	TO SEE DOCTOR IF . . .	
1. Name and age of child?	All children with rashes should be seen the same or next day.	
2. Please describe the rash and where it is located.	No further questions are necessary once an appointment has been given.	
3. How long has the rash been present?		

4. Are there any associated symptoms?
    Fever?
    Sore throat?
    Earache?
		○
		○
		○

5. Poison ivy or chickenpox	• Infected, complicated by swelling (p. ivy). • Located on eye or in severe pain (chickenpox). • signs of infection are present.	
6. Diaper rash.		☐

Stat		☆☆	**Same Day**	●
Same Session ASAP		☆	**Appointment (24–72 hrs.)**	☐
Same Session		○	**Appointment (4 days or more)**	■

High priority items are shaded

ADVICE

Under certain circumstances, as discussed under General Information, home management advice for specific rashes may be appropriate. Advice for these selected rashes is as follows:

Treatment of Plantar Warts with 40% Salicylic Acid Plaster

• Apply the plaster after a bath or shower.
• Cut the plaster to the exact outline of the wart. Do not apply the plaster to normal skin.
• Plaster will not remain attached to warts on the soles. Cover them with adhesive tape, using a strip of sufficient length to extend up the sides of the feet where it will be firmly attached.
• Leave plaster in place for 24 hrs. Remove prior to bath or shower and apply a fresh plaster afterward.

- If skin becomes irritated or uncomfortable, forego treatment for 2 or 3 days.
- Do not use plaster if wart appears infected. Call for an appointment.
- Parent should not expect wart to be gone in a manner of weeks. Stress that the wart might persist for months and that patience is needed.

Treatment of Poison Ivy or Chickenpox
- Apply calamine lotion with a cotton ball (poison ivy).
- Tub bath with either Alpha Keri bath oil or Aveeno oatmeal bath (2 cps added to tepid bath water).
- For itching, administer an antihistamine, Chlor-Trimeton (reduce dose if child becomes too drowsy). A prescription is not required.
- Cut fingernails as short as possible and keep clean.
- With chickenpox, use acetaminophen as needed for fever and for discomfort. No aspirin.

Uncomplicated Diaper Rash
- Bathe with warm water.
- Dry thoroughly with towel, or if available, use a blow-dryer 8–10 inches away from body and set on low heat to avoid burns.
- Leave diaper area exposed to air for prolonged periods of time (½–1 hr) during the day, such as during naps.
- Change diapers frequently. Avoid plastic pants.
- Apply thick coat of Vaseline or Desitin after each cleansing.

Age of Child

	Under 1 yr	*1–5 yrs*	*6–12 yrs*	*Over 12 yrs*
Chlor-Trimeton Syrup (2 mg/tsp) Tablet (4 mg/tab)	Not recommended unless specified by MD	½ tsp three or four times daily	1 tsp three or four times daily	2 tsp or 1 tab three times daily

CHAPTER **20**

Headache

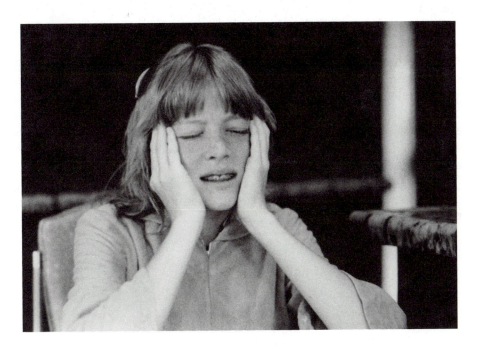

Headaches can be acute (of recent onset) or chronic and recurrent (long-standing). Most acute headaches are associated with infectious illnesses, like colds or influenza. Frequently, it is the fever itself that causes the headache. One of the most serious infections associated with headache is meningitis, an infection of the lining covering the brain and spinal canal. In meningitis, the child appears seriously ill, has a stiff neck, and is extremely irritable. In encephalitis, a viral brain infection, headache is often throbbing and the child's behavior and personality are abnormal. Whenever headache is accompanied by mental confusion, immediate medical care is urgently needed.

Chronic and recurring headaches are extremely common complaints among children. Perhaps the most common cause is stress and tension, reflecting the fast pace and lifestyle of today's children. The typical history of a tension headache is pain and pressure in the muscles at the base of the skull that occurs more frequently at the end of the day. The diagnosis of tension headache is one of exclusion, since headaches can be caused by any number of more serious medical problems. These include childhood migraine, sinus infections, dental problems, high blood pressure (commonly described as throbbing), and brain tumors, in which the headache often awakens the child from sleep and is worse after lying down. It may be associated with early morning vomiting, which relieves the pain.

Since all patients with headache need an examination, the role of the telephone assistant is to help decide upon the timing of the appointment. Any patient with an acute headache, or if the patient is acting ill or is in severe pain, needs to be seen right away. If the headache has been long-standing, if there has been no recent change in pattern, and if the child is in school and functioning normally, a future appointment is advisable. As with any problem, the earliest possible appointment should be arranged. If the level of parental anxiety is high, that alone should prompt an appointment as soon as possible.

Following is a chart offering decision guidelines. Questions in the left column correspond to suggested responses in the right column. High priority items are shaded.

TELEPHONE DECISION GUIDELINES
CHRONIC OR RECURRENT HEADACHE[a]

QUESTION	TO SEE DOCTOR IF . . .	
1. Name and age of child?		
2. How long have headaches been present?	Future appointment if duration is more than 1 month, child is not ill, and there are no serious associated symptoms.	○
3. Are there any associated symptoms: vomiting, stiff neck, difficulty with vision, recent behavior or personality change, or drowsiness?	Yes, see immediately.	☆☆
4. If vomiting is present, does it occur in the early morning?	Yes, schedule same day appointment.	●
5. Has there been a recent head injury?	Yes, schedule same day appointment.	●
6. How often do the headaches occur and are they getting worse or better? Are you treating with any medication now?	Schedule same day appointment if headaches are daily and the frequency and degree of pain are becoming worse and are unresponsive to treatment.	●
7. Does child appear ill?	Yes.	○
8. Does child have any other serious chronic medical disorder?	Yes, and there may be an association, schedule same day appointment.	●

Stat	☆☆	**Same Day**	●
Same Session ASAP	☆	**Appointment (24–72 hrs.)**	□
Same Session	○	**Appointment (4 days or more)**	■

High priority items are shaded

[a]This guideline is not applicable for headache of acute onset, or if it is associated with fever or upper respiratory infections. In this instance, use the relevant guideline for the specific problem.

CHAPTER 21

Burning and Frequency of Urination

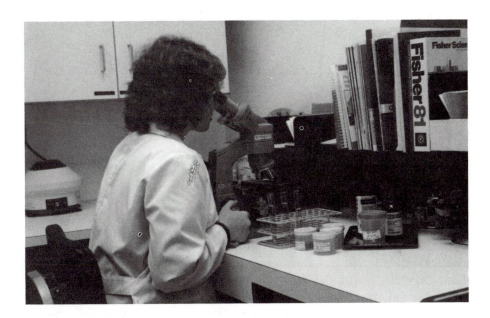

The complaint of burning (dysuria) and frequency of urination is much more common in females. A common cause is a vaginal infection, with or without a discharge, which irritates the urinary outlet. Bubble baths for children should be discouraged. Also, with pinworm infection, the worms may crawl from the anus to the vagina and irritate the vagina. Treatment for both the vaginitis as well as the pinworms is indicated. A more serious cause of dysuria and frequency is urinary tract infection.

URINARY TRACT INFECTION

Urinary tract infections (UTI) are one of the most common and important forms of bacterial infection in childhood. The urinary tract includes the

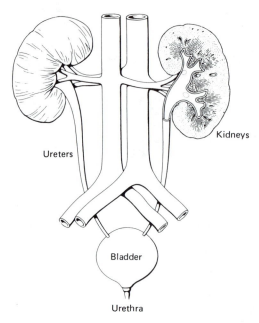

Figure 8

Schematic representation of the urinary tract.

kidneys, ureters, bladder, and urethra (Fig. 8). After the age of 1 year, UTI occurs ten times more commonly in females than in males. Symptoms can include the recent onset of bedwetting, abdominal pain, chronic diarrhea, chills, and fever, in addition to urinary burning and frequency. Some urinary tract infections cause little or no symptoms. *The urine culture is the critical diagnostic test.* The culture determines whether infection is present, what bacteria are causing the infection, and the best drugs with which to treat the infection.

Collecting Urine for the Urine Culture

Parents must be carefully instructed in the method for obtaining a clean-catch urine specimen at home. Thorough cleansing of the urethral opening is essential (Fig. 8). The middle of the stream, if possible, should be obtained in a sterile container. The urine should be refrigerated immediately and delivered to the office or laboratory *within 2 hours* or sooner after collection. A contaminated culture can be avoided by (1) proper cleansing, (2) proper collection, and (3) delivering the urine specimen promptly to the laboratory. The longer the delay, the more chance for contamination and therefore the need to repeat the collection.

Causes of Urinary Tract Infection

Approximately one-third of girls and the majority of boys who have a urinary tract infection will have a demonstrable cause for the infection:

1. *Obstruction*: a narrowing of the urinary tract in any of its locations.
2. *Reflux*: a back-up of urine from the bladder into the ureters.
3. *Pyelonephritis*: scarring of the kidney as a result of longstanding or recurrent infections.
4. *Anomalies*: abnormalities of the kidneys and urinary tract with which the child is born (an example is a horseshoe-shaped kidney).

There are, however, a large number of children whose urinary tracts appear normal by roentgenogram but nevertheless have recurrent UTI. The cause in these instances remains unknown.

Diagnostic Tests

To rule out obstruction, reflux, pyelonephritis, and anomalies, one or more of the following tests can be ordered by the physician *after the infection is cleared up.*

1. *Intravenous pyelogram* (IVP): A test in which dye is injected intravenously and then x-ray films are taken of the kidney and upper tracts.
2. *Sonogram*: A test using ultrasound that maps out the urinary tract structures without any injection of dye.
3. *Cystogram*: In this test, the child is catheterized and dye is introduced into the bladder. As the child urinates, x-ray films are taken of the lower tract and bladder. In this way, reflux and bladder neck obstruction are diagnosed.

If an anatomical abnormality is demonstrated, a referral to a urologist is appropriate.

PAIN ON URINATION IN THE MALE

Urinary tract infection is much less common in boys. A negative urinalysis and urine culture rules out UTI in boys who complain of dysuria. Local irritation at the tip of the penis is a more common cause, sometimes associated with masturbation. In adolescents, infection of the urethra by a variety of bacteria is a major cause of dysuria. Venereal disease should be ruled out by appropriate tests. A discharge from the penis does not always accompany the infection. All males with dysuria should be given a same-day appointment.

FREQUENCY WITHOUT DYSURIA

One should always be on the alert for the symptoms of diabetes when a child has frequent painless urination. Symptoms include urinating large volumes of urine frequently, intense thirst, increased appetite, and weight loss. There also may be the recent onset of bedwetting. All patients with suggestive histories should be seen as soon as possible for a physical examination and urinalysis.

Following is a chart offering decision guidelines. Questions in the left column correspond to suggested responses in the right column. High priority items are shaded.

BURNING AND FREQUENCY OF URINATION

QUESTION	TO SEE DOCTOR IF . . .	
1. Name and age of child.		
2. How long has child had pain on urination?	More than 24 hours.	●
3. Is fever present?	Yes.	●
4. Is there any sign of local redness or irritation at the tip of the penis (or of the vagina)?	Home advice appropriate.	
5. Does the child appear ill?	Yes.	○
6. Has child had a urinary tract infection in past?	Yes.	●
7. Is frequency present without pain?	Obtain UA/UC if UA negative, see 1–2 days.	□ ●
8. Is there (if female) a vaginal discharge present?	Yes.	●
9. Is there (if female) itching of the rectum present?	Yes.	●
10. Does the child bathe with bubble bath?	Advise to discontinue bubble bath. Parents should bring in a urine specimen for urinalysis and urine culture.	

Stat	☆☆	**Same Day**	●
Same Session ASAP	☆	**Appointment (24–72 hrs.)**	□
Same Session	○	**Appointment (4 days or more)**	■

High priority items are shaded

ADVICE

If there is no fever, the child appears well, and mild symptoms have been present for less than 24 hrs:

- Bring a sterile urine specimen to the office for urinalysis and urine culture.

- Place child in sitz bath of plain warm water for relief of pain.

- Child may void directly into water.

- Place Vaseline or A and D Ointment on the area of irritation at tip of penis if redness is visible.

- Call office in 24 hrs for urine culture results and to report effect of treatment on symptoms. If child is worse or if urine test is abnormal, schedule appointment for same day.

If there is a history of frequency, inquire about the presence of increased thirst, increased appetite, and weight loss—the classical triad for diabetes. Also, the increased urination is sometimes manifested by the recent onset of bedwetting. An appointment should be given as soon as possible. If there is no appointment available until later in the day and the child is not ill, parents can be instructed to bring in a urinalysis immediately to determine if diabetes is present. If it is negative, there is no sense of urgency. If it is positive, the patient should be called for an immediate appointment. This arrangement, of course, depends on how close to the office or clinic the family lives, and their available transportation.

Collecting a Proper Urine Specimen at Home

- **Child should be completely unclothed (pants and panties), and sit straddling the toilet.**

- **Wash genitalia gently with soap and water.**

- **Try to catch middle of stream if at all possible.**

- **Urinate into a small jar which, with the cover, has been boiled for 20 min and then air-cooled.**

- **Specimen should be refrigerated immediately and brought to the office as soon as possible (within 2 hrs).**

CHAPTER **22**

 # Poisonings

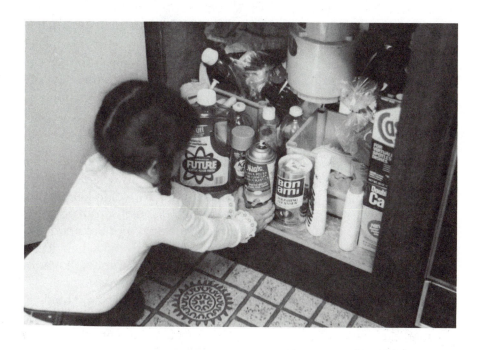

Accidental poisoning of children is a major, year-round concern. Accidents and poisonings in the United States account for the largest number of deaths among children—more than the next seven causes of fatalities combined. It is estimated that 500,000 children in the United States will be victims of accidental poisoning in the next 12 months and that 500 to 1,000 of these children will die. Children are by nature curious and love to experiment. The following features of accidental childhood poisoning may be of interest:

1. Ninety percent of all cases reported involve children under 5 years of age.

2. Most of these ingestions occur in the presence of an adult and in the late afternoon.

3. The most hazardous location for accidental poisoning in your home is the kitchen (look beneath your sink).

4. Aspirin, household detergents and bleach, and vitamins lead the list of poisons. Tranquilizer poisoning is on the increase.

5. Frequently ingested substances are drain cleaners, such as Drano and Liquid-plumr, turpentine, kerosene, furniture polish, paints, and many other household preparations.

6. Aspirin—a frequent cause of accidental poisoning in this country—can, in large doses, cause deep, rapid breathing, dehydration, fever, convulsions, coma, and death.

7. Ingestion of vitamin preparations that also contain iron can cause vomiting of blood, diarrhea, coma, shock, and death. Countless other ingested substances are life threatening.

You can take simple, but major, steps to eliminate the danger of accidental ingestion of poisons by "poison-proofing" your home.

1. All household products and medications *must* be kept out of sight and reach of children and should be kept in a locked cabinet or closet. When you are using a medication, be careful to keep it out of the reach of small children. *Two-thirds of poisonings from household medications occur because the medicine was not returned to its usual storage place.* Medicine should be discarded when it is no longer needed. A medicine chest filled with half-empty leftover bottles is dangerous. Clean out your medicine cabinet periodically. The safest way to dispose of unused or discarded medicine, liquids and pills, is to flush them down the toilet. Bottles that contained liquid medicine should be rinsed with water before they are tossed in the wastebasket.

2. Medicine should be called "medicine"—and not candy. Candy-flavored medications present the greatest temptation. Candy-flavored vitamins belong in the garbage disposal, not in the medicine cabinet.

3. Medications should be kept apart from other household products and in their original, properly labeled containers. *Always check the label and dosage before administering a medication.*

4. When storing household products, such as bleaches, polishes, and insecticides, avoid the use of easily accessible cabinets.

5. Request the safest medicine containers (palm and turn) whenever possible.

If, despite all precautions, a child does ingest a medication or other household substance, parents should call their physician for advice on the potential danger and the need for further therapy. It might even be better to call the Poison Control Center at _____ (fill in telephone number).

When a parent is advised to bring a child who has ingested a substance to the office, they should be instructed to bring the original container so that the ingredients can be verified.

SYRUP OF IPECAC

Parents can be instructed to administer Ipecac Syrup to their child. Ipeca Syrup is a reliable emetic—that is, a substance that induces vomiting. The proper dosage for a child 1 to 4 years of age is 3 teaspoonfuls given after drinking 4 to 8 ounces of warm water. *This is to be given only on instruction from your physician or poison control center.* Vomiting will usually occur within 15 to 20 minutes after the administration of the ipecac. *Ipecac Syrup should never be used and vomiting should not be induced after the ingestion of lye, petroleum products, or other corrosive substances, or in the very young or stuporous child.* While it is advantageous for all families with children under the age of 5 years to have syrup of ipecac in the home, please *remember it is to be administered only on instruction from your physician and stored safely locked up.*

Following is a chart offering decision guidelines. Questions in the left column correspond suggested responses in the right column. High priority items are shaded.

POISONING

QUESTION	TO SEE DOCTOR IF . . .	
1. What is name, address, age, and phone number of patient, and what was ingested (details in question no. 8)?		
2. What is patient's status? (i.e., alert, drowsy)	Lethargic, drowsy, hyperirritable, obvious lesions, such as mouth or skin burns, or any symptoms resulting from ingestion, such as vomiting or abdominal pain.	☆☆
3. How much time has elapsed since ingestion?	**a)** Time of ingestion is unknown. **b)** Time of ingestion is over 4 hrs.	☆☆
4. What information is available on the label of ingested substance? (i.e., antidotes, first aid, etc.)^a		
5. Has Poison Control been called?	Poison Control Center so advises (based on potential toxicity).	
6. What is availability of syrup of ipecac at home?	None available at home, and emesis is indicated.	
7. Has vomiting already taken place?	Vomiting was of a corrosive or petroleum distallate (*no* syrup of ipecac).	☆☆
8. How much was taken?		
9. What is weight of child?^b		
10. What is nature of substance ingested (trade and/or generic): plant, corrosive, paint thinner, furniture polish, nail polish remover or drug.	Ingestion is of: **a)** *Most pills* (i.e., iron vitamins, sleeping medications, barbiturates, aspirin, *any* unknown pills. Note: Some pills (antihistamines, compazine, barbiturates) will have antivomiting	

Stat	☆☆	**Same Day**	●
Same Session ASAP	☆	**Appointment (24–72 hrs.)**	□
Same Session	○	**Appointment (4 days or more)**	■

High priority items are shaded

QUESTION	TO SEE DOCTOR IF . . .	
	effects, making syrup of ipecac less effective. **b)** *All narcotics* and *tranquilizers* (methadone, tricyclics, like imipramine, amitriptyline). (Tofranil, Elavil) **c)** All plants, seeds, berries, wild mushrooms. **d)** All *insecticides, rodenticides* (rat poisons) **e)** All corrosives (strong acids, alkalies, i.e., lye) **f)** *Hydrocarbons* (kerosene, paint thinners, turpentine, and furniture polish).	

Stat	☆☆	**Same Day**	●
Same Session ASAP	☆	**Appointment (24–72 hrs.)**	□
Same Session	○	**Appointment (4 days or more)**	■

ADVICE

The patient's name, address, and phone number are especially important to obtain because many parents will neglect to provide it in their haste and panic.

If the time of ingestion is unknown, do *not* delay at home to induce vomiting (even if indicated). Bring child immediately to office. Follow immediate first aid measures at home, then bring child to clinic.

If poison control center has been called, follow their immediate suggestions first, then bring child for evaluation.

If ingestion was of pills, nonpetroleum substances, noncorrosives, may induce vomiting with syrup of ipecac.

Induce vomiting with one tbsp of syrup of ipecac after giving 4 to 8 oz of warm water. Repeat in 20 min if vomiting has not occurred. (See note re: antiemetic pills, liquids). Certain ingestions do not require a visit.

For corrosives (lye) or hydrocarbons (kerosene, furniture polish) do not induce vomiting. Bring child to office or clinic immediately.

In a true emergency, an ambulance should be summoned.

Always have parents bring in the container and label containing any pertinent information on the nature of the substance.

Instances in which ingestions may be managed conservatively at home: (There is no immediate need to bring the child into the office unless symptoms are present. Case should be reported to the physician.)

- *Coins* and smooth metallic objects (provided no vomiting, abdominal pain, coughing, respiratory distress, or cyanosis is present). If object is lead, child should be seen at once.

- Small nonmetallic toys and parts of toys (with above exceptions).

- *Cosmetics* (powders, creams—if nail polish remover or hair dye, child should be brought in).

- *Clorox* and *bleaches* (may cause oral and esophageal burns if in concentrated form. Cases should be judged on an individual basis).

- *Mercury* (metallic) from broken thermometers.

- *Aspirin,* when dosage is low (less than 100 mg/kg) and/or elasped time is 1 hour or less, and syrup of ipecac is available in the home (e.g., 6–10 baby aspirin in a 30 lb. child when no symptoms are present).

- Vitamin pills that *definitely* contain no iron.

- Birth control pills (under 6 pills).

CHAPTER 23

Animal Bites

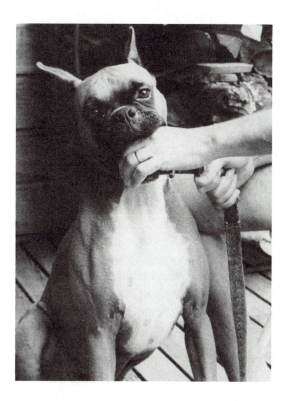

The potential hazards of animal bites include infection with rabies, tetanus, and other bacterial agents causing local skin infections, and the emotional trauma to the child as a result of the frightening experience.

Rabies is an acute viral infection that spreads via peripheral nerves into the brain causing a highly fatal encephalitis or brain infection. According to data from the Communicable Disease Center, animal rabies is on the increase in the United States. The rabies virus is transmitted between animals in the infected saliva of a biting, warm-blooded animal. There are over 40 species of animals in the world that can be infected with rabies. Specific information about which animals have been infected with rabies in any given location can be obtained from the state health department, along with a detailed report of the types and numbers of animal bites in general for that state. The reports usually categorize data according to bites by common house pets (cats, dogs, hamsters, rabbits); animals of agriculture (horses, calves); primates (monkeys); wild rodents (chipmunks, ground hogs, mice, rats, squirrels); wild animals (bats, ferrets, raccoons, skunks); amphibians and reptiles (snakes, turtles, alligators); and various miscellaneous animals, like spiders, camels, and crabs. In most instances, rodent bites can be assumed to be free of the threat of rabies. These lists are very useful in describing the extent of the animal bite problem in any given area.

Fortunately, human infection is rare. Symptoms can occur in as short as 3 days, or as long as 6 to 9 months, depending on the amount of virus introduced into the wound (as in an extensive or vicious bite), and also on the abundance of nerve supply at the wound site. Rabies virus can be present in a dog's saliva for 2 to 7 days before the onset of symptoms, but bats can be infected for more than a year without developing signs of illness. Therefore, it is important to note that some animals can transmit the disease at a time when there are no symptoms. When dogs develop symptoms of rabies, death usually occurs in 4 to 5 days, making the 10-day observation period a valuable component of management. All bat bites should be considered as an exposure to rabies. The diagnosis of rabies is based on specific laboratory tests performed on brain and salivary gland tissue, together with a clinical evaluation of the biting animal and the circumstances surrounding the incident. The prompt apprehension and careful observation of the biting animal is mandatory. If bats, skunks, racoons, and other wild animals are not captured, they must be assumed to be rabid. If captured, they should be sacrificed and the brain examined for rabies. Dog vaccination and animal control programs are of the utmost importance for effective rabies prevention. Fortunately, there is a new vaccine that is safer, more effective, and requires many fewer injections than the older vaccine.

Local skin infections can be prevented by thorough soap and water cleansing of the wound. If the wound is extensive or deep, then an appointment for an examination, as soon as possible, should be given. The risk of tetanus is present, so immunization status should be reviewed.

TETANUS IMMUNIZATION

A child has completed his primary series of tetanus shots for protection against lockjaw after he has received four doses, the last dose usually given at the 18-month well-baby visit. A booster dose is administered at between 4 and 6 years of age, and then every 10 years.

After an animal bite or a cut, tetanus shots are advised:

- If more than 10 years after the last shot.
- If more than 5 years after the last shot and the wound is very dirty and contaminated.
- If a child is under 6 years old and has not finished the complete four-dose series.
- If a child has never been immunized, series should be started and completed.

Following is a chart offering decision guidelines. Questions in the left column correspond to suggested responses in the right column. High priority items are shaded.

ANIMAL BITES

QUESTION	SEE DOCTOR IF . . .	
1. What is name, address, and phone number of patient?	Unprovoked bites by wild animals, which would normally shy away from human contact, are at highest risk for rabies. These children should be examined.	☆
2. What were the circumstances of the animal bite? When did it occur? What kind of animal bit the child? Was it a wild animal or a household pet? If a pet dog, has it been immunized for rabies? Is the animal available for observation?	*Child is bitten by a bat, skunk, fox, raccoon, or monkey, child must be seen immediately.* The animal cannot be located within a few hrs, the child should be brought in and the circumstances reviewed by the physician. Large lacerations requiring sutures, lacerations of the face or hand area, should be seen by a surgeon.	☆
3. Was the skin broken? Where are the bites? How severe is the injury?	Bites appearing infected or on the face should also be seen in the office.	☆
4. What is the child's tetanus immunization status?	No tetanus immunization within 10 years, child should have booster (assuming primary series is complete), or if it has been more than 5 years and the wound is very dirty. This can wait up to 24 hours, if necessary.	
Stat ☆☆ **Same Session ASAP** ☆ **Same Session** ○	**Same Day** ● **Appointment (24–72 hrs.)** ☐ **Appointment (4 days or more)** ■	
High priority items are shaded		

ADVICE

Every effort should be made to locate the animal so that its health may be determined. The health department should be notified about animal bites so that appropriate investigation may be made (pet dogs will not be taken away from their owners because of such a report).

Telephone #: _____County Health Department (fill in phone number)

Nights and Weekends #: _____ Police Department

If the skin is not broken or if there is a scratch, the wound should be cleaned with soap and water and observed for infection.

Uninfected bites by small household pets, such as mice, hamsters, and gerbils, are not at risk for rabies and need not be seen. The same advice applies for most rodents, including squirrels.

CHAPTER **24**

Insect Bites and Stings

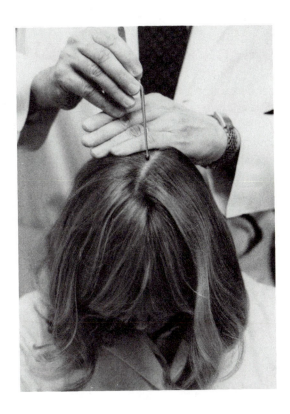

Insect bites and children go together with good weather and outdoor play. Reactions to the bite or sting of an insect are painful because of the chemical material injected into the skin, but usually are not dangerous. Symptoms can be local (confined to the area of the bite) or generalized (spreading to other parts of the body). Generalized reactions can be dangerous because of an overwhelming allergic reaction leading to shock. Although this type of reaction is rare, the potential danger of an insect bite should always be kept in mind.

LOCAL REACTIONS

The majority of insect bites and Hymenoptera (wasp, bee, hornet, yellow jacket, and ant) stings are not serious and usually require no special care.

129

If the stinger remains in the skin, it should be extracted by scraping it off with a knife blade or fingernail. If the stinger cannot be seen, it most likely is not there. There may be marked local swelling which occasionally involves an entire hand or foot. Itching, burning, and stinging are common after a bite. Pressure with an ice cube relieves the pain and swelling. Topical application of calamine lotion or an antihistamine taken by mouth can be used for further relief.

GENERALIZED REACTION

When a generalized reaction occurs, there can be a dry cough, a sense of chest or throat constriction, swelling and itching around the eyes, hives, wheezing, pallor, and a sense of anxiety. Symptoms occur within the first few minutes following the sting. In some cases, symptoms could progress to life-threatening shock, which requires immediate emergency treatment.

Once it has been determined that a child has had a generalized rather than local reaction, prevention is of prime importance. Since the peak sting season is from April to October (when insects are naturally more aggressive) careful inspection of home and grounds should be made to detect and carefully eliminate nests. Perfumes, hair spray, scented skin lotions, and other scented cosmetics should be avoided. Going barefoot invites problems. Insect repellants, such as Off, should be used on outings. Following a generalized reaction, a program of desensitization or "allergy shots" should be considered. Hyposensitization should not be depended on to totally prevent a serious reaction. For this reason, a bee sting emergency kit is prescribed to keep in the home after proper instruction is given in its use.

Tick Bites

Tick bites may be a problem, depending on where people live. A small percentage (1–5%) of wood ticks may become infected with an organism (*Rickettsia*), which is the agent that causes Rocky Mountain Spotted Fever (RMSF), so named because the first case came from the Bitterroot Valley of Montana. In fact, there is no geographical boundary. The number of cases in Maryland, Delaware, and Virginia ranks among the highest in the nation.

The transmission of RMSF is from animal to man by way of the wood or dog tick. Animals, like squirrels, chipmunks, weasels, and jack rabbits, carry the Rickettsia germ but do not become ill. Most cases occur in the summer because of the increased chance of encountering ticks in the woods. The incubation period varies from 1 to 8 days. The illness starts with nonspecific symptoms, such as headache, fever, irritability, or lethargy. A characteristic rash appears 2 to 6 days after the onset of fever. It is a salmon-colored flat rash that usually begins on the extremities (wrist, ankle, palms, and soles) and spreads toward the trunk. There frequently is a throbbing headache and marked muscular aching. There is a history of tick bite in only half of the cases, so a negative exposure history does not rule out RMSF. If antibiotics are not begun early in suspicious cases, the disease can be fatal.

Fortunately, the likelihood of getting RMSF after a tick bite is very low. Prevention is helped by early removal of the tick, since attachment of the tick for several hours is required for the introduction of infected material into the human. It is very important to avoid crushing the tick while removing it, since infected material could be squeezed from the tick into the bite wound. While on outings and hikes, periodic tick checks can help reduce the risk of infection. The scalp, neck, wrists, and ankles are favorite spots for ticks. Since one cannot feel the tick embedding into the skin, these areas should be inspected carefully.

LYME DISEASE

Another tick-borne illness, Lyme disease, was originally described in 1977. It was so named because the first identified outbreak of the illness clustered, geographically, around Lyme, Connecticut. It is now recognized that it can occur anywhere. Lyme disease is a multisystem disorder which can affect primarily the skin (rash), the joints (arthritis), the nervous system (meningo-encephalitis, Bell's palsy), and the heart (myopericarditis). The causative agent which is carried by the tick is a type of bacterium called a spirochete. One clue may be a distinctive rash (erythema chronicum migrans), which begins at the site of the tick bite and gradually becomes larger with an area of central clearing. Patients who report tick bites should be asked if there is a red spot around the bite, and if any of the joints hurt or are swollen. There is also a potential risk to the fetus if the pregnant mother contracts Lyme disease. Fortunately, the illness responds to antibiotic treatment. Early diagnosis and treatment are the keys to reducing complications.

Spider Bites

Any child bitten by a spider should be seen as soon as possible. The two most dangerous spiders in North America are the black widow and brown recluse.

Following is a chart offering decision guidelines. Questions in the left column correspond to suggested responses in the right column. High priority items are shaded.

INSECT BITES

QUESTION	SEE DOCTOR IF . . .	
1. Age, name of child, and when bite occurred.		
2. Did you see what bit the child?	Yes, if bitten by spider, scorpion, or centipede.	☆
3. Is the area around the bite red, swollen, or itchy?		
4. Has child had a serious allergic reaction to an insect bite before?	Yes.	☆☆
5. Is there any difficulty breathing, lightheadedness, swelling around eyes, or widespread rash all over body?	Yes (immediately).	☆☆
6. If child was bitten longer than 24 hrs ago—is reaction to bite getting redder or more swollen?	Yes.	○
7. Does bite look infected?	Yes.	●
If Insect Is a Tick **8.** Is tick embedded in skin?	See tick removal advice.	
9. Is child acting ill?	Yes.	○
10. If tick bite was more than 24 hrs ago, is there any fever, headache, rash, or muscle aches?	Yes.	○
11. Does bite look infected?	Yes.	●

Stat	☆☆	**Same Day**	●
Same Session ASAP	☆	**Appointment (24–72 hrs.)**	□
Same Session	○	**Appointment (4 days or more)**	■

High priority items are shaded

ADVICE

Cold compresses or ice can be applied to reduce the swelling. If bite is very itchy, an antihistamine can be used orally. Use emergency kit if available in home.

Use emergency kit if previously instructed in use, or take an antihistamine right away. Do not delay.

Tick Removal Advice

- Cover tick with nail polish remover or alcohol.
- Grasp body of tick firmly with a tweezer and remove head from skin by using steady gentle traction.
- Do *not* use match or cigarette.

CHAPTER **25**

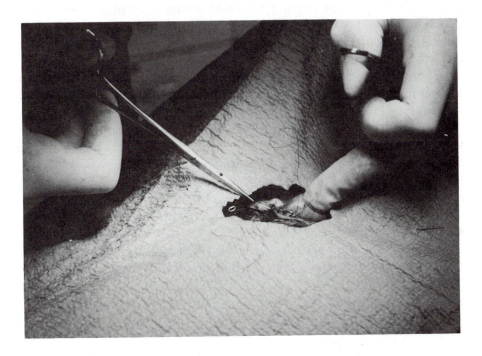

Puncture Wounds, Lacerations, and Abrasions

Puncture wounds and lacerations are among the most common injuries that are reported by parents. In the case of both of these types of trauma, the key considerations are (1) an assessment of the need for repair or sutures; (2) whether there has been damage to adjacent structures, like the eye or a joint; (3) the risk of infection at the site of the cut or lymph glands; (4) risk of tetanus; and (5) control of bleeding. If bleeding from a cut does occur, it usually can be stopped by gentle, firm pressure. The degree of bleeding from a small cut, particularly on the forehead or in the mouth and tongue, can be misleading, since the amount of blood may be out of proportion to the size of the laceration because of the rich blood vessel supply in these areas. Parents should be instructed to blot the wound dry and inspect the bleeding site in order to assess the wound more objectively. The location of the injury also can give a clue as to the nature of the injury. For example, cuts around the genitals raise the suspicion of child abuse. As indicated in the guidelines, tetanus can infect any laceration or puncture wound, so it is important to make sure that the child's tetanus shots are up-to-date. Tetanus is not a concern if there is just an abrasion. Generally, a thorough cleansing will clean the wound of debris and lessen the risk of infection.

Small puncture wounds, superficial cuts, and scrapes (abrasions) can be treated effectively at home. However, if there is any question about whether sutures will be needed, the child should be examined as soon as possible. The longer the delay between the injury and the repair, the greater the risk of infection. If there are severe multiple lacerations with uncontrollable bleeding (unable to stop after 10 minutes of direct pressure), particularly when there has been a serious accident, it is advisable to instruct the parent to call an ambulance to transport the child to the nearest hospial emergency room.

Abrasions are areas of scraped-off skin which are commonly caused when children "skin" themselves after a fall from a bicycle or skateboard onto a rough surface-like concrete or gravel. When the abrasion is on the side of the buttock or thigh, parents may refer to it as a strawberry. Most abrasions are effectively treated at home by proper cleansing and observation for signs of infection. If the abrasion appears infected, the child should be examined.

Following is a chart offering decision guidelines. Questions in the left column correspond to suggested responses in the right column. High priority items are shaded.

PUNCTURE WOUNDS, LACERATIONS, AND ABRASIONS

QUESTION	TO SEE DOCTOR IF . . .	
1. Name and age of child.	Under one year.	
2. Is the wound bleeding?	Bleeding will not stop.	☆☆
3. When and how did it occur? (e.g., was nail rusty or clean; inside or outside of home?)	Wound is contaminated. (Check immunization status)	☆☆
4. Is it a very deep puncture wound?	Yes.	☆
5. Is there foreign material visible in the wound?	Yes.	☆
6. Are there any signs of local infection in the area? Redness Swelling Red streaks extending from the wound Discharge or pus draining from wound	There is any suspicion of infection.	○
7. Did your child have the complete primary series of tetanus shots? (3 or more)	No.	
8. When was last booster?	Needs a booster.	●
9. Have you cleansed the wound thoroughly?	Advise for home treatment.	
Laceration **1.** How did it occur and where is the cut located on the body?	Site is around eye, in mouth, genitals, over a joint, or on the face.	☆
2. Is the cut still bleeding?	Bleeding will not stop after 10 min of direct, firm pressure.	☆
3. Does the cut look bad; is it gaping or split open? Is it jagged or deep?	There is any laceration that is more than a small scratch, the child should be seen to determine the need for stitches.	○

All questions regarding infection and tetanus are the same as for puncture wound (6–9).

Stat	☆☆	**Same Day**	●
Same Session ASAP	☆	**Appointment (24–72 hrs.)**	□
Same Session	○	**Appointment (4 days or more)**	■

High priority items are shaded

ADVICE

Apply direct pressure firmly for 10 min to stop bleeding.

Tetanus Shots are Advised for Wounds:

- If more than 10 yrs after the last shot.
- If more than 5 yrs after the last shot if the wound is very dirty and contaminated, or if it is a deep puncture.
- If a child is under 6 yrs old and has not finished the complete 4-dose series.
- If a child has never been immunized, series should be started and completed.

Wash the Wound[a] Very Thoroughly as Follows:

- Flush with cool water running from tap. If the area cannot be held under the faucet, soak it in a basin of slightly cool water.
- Scrub gently with soap and water, using a soft washcloth, and rinse.
- Apply an antiseptic, like betadine, 3% hydrogen peroxide, or mercurochrome.
- Dry and cover with band-aid or sterile gauze if cut is in an area that is likely to get dirty. Use Telfa non-sticking dressing if it is a large abrasion.
- Observe daily for any signs of local infection or signs of illness.

Apply firm pressure with a clean cloth and control bleeding before starting out for the office.

Same as for puncture wound and abrasion.

[a]The above advice is appropriate for puncture wounds and abrasions.

CHAPTER 26

Head Injury

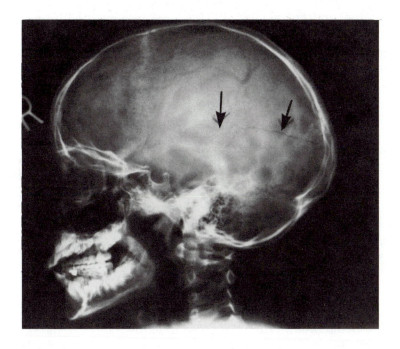

It is important for the telephone care assistant to be aware that the physician's role in evaluating children with head injury is to decide on the necessity for consultation with a neurosurgeon and hospitalization. Very few children require this, but a careful evaluation in the office and very close follow-up at home by the parent are essential elements of management. The complaint of head injury is a very common one since very few children escape injuring their heads at some time in their lives.

Definitions are in order. Not all head injuries are concussions. Injury to the brain can occur in several ways, the concussion being the most common. A concussion is a form of closed head injury in which there is a transient loss of consciousness, and strange behavior or mental confusion followed by gradual recovery. Not all children with concussions lose consciousness. On some occasions, the major symptoms of a concussion may be temporary loss of vision, pallor, listlessness, memory loss, and/or vomiting. Symptoms may persist for many hours or be very transient.

Very few children require hospitalization. More severe head injuries, such as the contusion, or frank bleeding into the brain, as with a subdural or epidural hematoma, are extremely serious. The disturbed mental status in these conditions is more profound, and there are deficits of neurological function. Frequently the child has been in a serious accident and there are signs of multiple trauma to other parts of the body, such as fractures and internal abdominal injuries. These children must be hospitalized immediately.

The more common complaint for which most parents call the office is that their child has fallen and hit his or her head. If the fall was a significant one, it is best to bring the child into the office for an examination. If the fall was trivial and the child is acting fine, with no symptoms of concussion, it is appropriate to explain what signs and symptoms should be watched for at home, with instructions to call back if there is a significant change. The most important factor in evaluating the effects of head injury is what happens to the child over the course of time. Initially, it is common for mild symptoms to occur, such as pallor or a few episodes of vomiting; it is what develops after these initial symptoms that must be observed closely. Skull x-ray films are of no help in this regard. The presence of a skull fracture in most instances will not influence management. Conversely, the absence of a skull fracture does not rule out the possibility of a serious complication. Close observation is essential in either case, and good parental supervision at home is critical.

A bump or bruise on the head following injury represents bleeding into the skin (hematoma). When it is present on the forehead, the skin should be anticipated to undergo a color change—purple to yellow—and sometimes spread into the spaces around the eyes. Resolution of the bruise occurs in about 7 to 10 days. If the history of trauma is suspicious of child abuse, the child should be given an appointment as quickly as possible.

Following is a chart offering decision guidelines. Questions in the left column correspond to suggested responses in the right column. High priority items are shaded.

HEAD INJURY

	QUESTION	TO SEE DOCTOR IF . . .	
1.	Name and age of patient?		
2.	When did injury occur?		
3.	Did you see injury? How did it happen?	A high fall, automobile accident, or a strong blow. Also, if description raises suspicion of child abuse.	☆☆
4.	Has there been a convulsion? Loss of consciousness?	The child is convulsing or has been unconscious for longer than a few sec, an ambulance should be called. (911 or local emergency no.)	☆☆
5.	Is child acting normally?	*All children with any positive symptoms (questions 5–11) need to be seen as soon as possible.*	☆
6.	Has there been any mental confusion or strange behavior? Vomiting? Loss of vision? Pallor? Lethargy? Momentary loss of consciousness?		☆
7.	Has there been any discharge of blood or fluid from the nose or ears?		☆
8.	Does child have a headache?		☆
9.	Has there been any fever or stiff neck since the injury?		☆
10.	Has child had a head injury in the past?		☆
11.	Is there evidence of any other injury? Laceration? Abrasion? Abdominal pain? Failure to use arm or leg?		☆

Stat	☆☆	**Same Day**	●
Same Session ASAP	☆	**Appointment (24–72 hrs.)**	□
Same Session	○	**Appointment (4 days or more)**	■

High priority items are shaded

ADVICE

If injury was not witnessed by parent, ask if anyone else saw the fall, for example, a teacher at school.

If child is acting normally, and there were no symptoms of concussion, and if the injury was slight, the child can be observed at home for any of the following:

- Severe or increasing headache.
- Persistent or recurrent vomiting (more than three times).
- Dizziness or unsteadiness.
- Excessive or persistent drowsiness.
- Slurred speech.
- Clear or bloody discharge from nose or ears.
- Unequal pupil (black part of eye) size.
- Child may be sleepy after the injury. Allow nap but awaken 1 hr later to reevaluate and to make sure behavior is normal.
- Aspirin can be used for relief of headache or for the local pain of a bruise.
- Awaken child during the night at midnight and at 3 A.M. and 6 A.M. to make sure he or she is arousable and acting normally.

CHAPTER **27**

Strains and Sprains

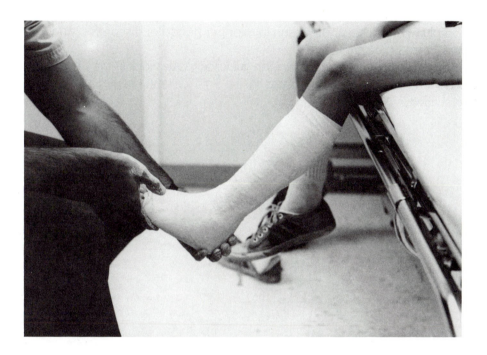

Minor orthopedic trauma prompts a large number of phone calls to the pediatrician or family practitioner. The majority of these injuries involve muscle strains and ligamentous sprains, usually involving the knee and ankle, and fractures. Whenever there are a large number of adolescents involved in sports, the incidence of injury will be even greater.

Muscle strains usually are quite painful but not serious. The role of the telephone assistant is to rule out the possibility that the strain is actually not something else, like a fracture or joint problem. In most cases of strained muscles, the child can trace the injury to starting a new sport or overexerting himself or herself in gym class. If there is any doubt, the child should be examined. If there is a clear-cut explanation for the muscle strain, telephone care management with heat, aspirin, rest, and observation should remedy the situation in a short time.

Sprains are more serious and represent damage to the ligaments that attach to the bones of the joint. Ligaments surrounding any joint can be stretched in a mild sprain, torn or even separated in a more severe injury.

Sprains are produced by accidents that force the joint, such as the ankle and knee, into an abnormal position. The amount of pain and the degree of swelling can be comparable to that seen in a fracture.

Treatment of a sprain will depend on the extent of injury. For mild sprains, ICE, or *ice*, *compression*, and *elevation*, are helpful and the sprain usually is resolved within a few days. More severe sprains may require casting, crutches, or in the extreme cases, surgery. All but the most minor sprains should be examined, since failure to treat the sprain properly at the onset could result in a longer period of discomfort and less satisfactory outcome later on.

Following is a chart offering decision guidelines. Questions in the left column correspond to suggested responses in the right column. High priority items are shaded.

STRAINS

QUESTION	TO SEE DOCTOR IF . . .	
1. Name and age of child?		
2. What part of body was injured?		
3. When did injury occur?	More than 3 days ago.	●
4. How did the injury occur?	There is pain and no clear-cut history of muscle strain.	
5. Is there joint swelling?	Yes.	●
6. Is the area red, warm, or swollen?	Yes.	●
7. Is there any fever?	Yes.	●
8. Is pain severe?	Yes.	●
9. Does the child appear ill?	Yes.	●

Stat	☆☆	**Same Day**		●
Same Session ASAP	☆	**Appointment (24–72 hrs.)**		□
Same Session	○	**Appointment (4 days or more)**		■

High priority items are shaded

ADVICE

If there is a clear-cut history of a pulled or strained muscle, and there are no complicating factors, home management can be planned as follows:

• Rest.

• Heat (heating pad, hot water bag) for 15 min. four times a day until improved as needed.

• Aspirin for pain.

• Call back if symptoms worsen, do not improve, or if pain persists after 3 days of treatment.

TELEPHONE DECISION GUIDELINES
SPRAINS

QUESTION	TO SEE DOCTOR IF . . .	
1. Name and age of child?		
2. What joint is sprained?		
3. How did injury occur?		
4. Is joint red, hot, or swollen?	Yes.	☆
5. Is child in much pain when joint is moved?	Yes.	○
6. Is there any fever?	Yes.	○
7. Does child appear ill?	Yes.	○

Stat	☆☆	**Same Day**	●
Same Session ASAP	☆	**Appointment (24–72 hrs.)**	☐
Same Session	○	**Appointment (4 days or more)**	■

High priority items are shaded

ADVICE

All painful joints (knee, shoulder, elbow, back, neck, wrist, hip, hands, and feet) should be examined. The one exception is a minimal twist of the ankle unaccompanied by swelling, which is only slightly uncomfortable, and the parent is not anxious. In that instance, home management can be advised as follows:

- Wrap a plastic bag filled with ice in a towel and place over outside of joint for 20 minutes.

- Compress ankle by wrapping an ace bandage around the joint. Wrap the bandage from the bottom of the foot up, making the first wind toward the outside of the foot. Do not stretch bandage or make too tight. Foot should feel comfortable after wrapped. May keep on as long as bandage helps.

- Elevate foot.

- Aspirin for pain.

- Gradually increase use of foot.

- Call back if not improving.

CHAPTER **28**

 # Nosebleed

Nosebleeds are very common in young children. Although the experience can be frightening, particularly since it often occurs at night, a nosebleed rarely causes severe blood loss. The telephone assessment of this complaint has three purposes. One, it is important to instruct parents in the proper way to stop the bleeding. Second, it is necessary to make sure that there is no serious underlying bleeding disorder that caused the nosebleed, such as thrombocytopenic (low platelets) purpura, leukemia, or hemophilia. Fortunately, these bleeding disorders are very rare, and are determined easily by asking a few simple questions about the past and family history. Third, parents need to be instructed in what to look for after the acute bleed is over, as a guideline follow-up to insure that there are not repeated small bleeds over a long period of time. This could lead to enough chronic blood loss to result in anemia.

The lining of the septum of the nose contains many tiny blood vessels. As a result of local irritation from dryness or sneezing from a cold or allergy, these tiny vessels may break and bleed. Foreign bodies in the nose also can cause bleeding, often with an associated malodorous discharge of pus. Commonly, nosebleeds may follow injury, nose blowing or picking, and nasal infections. Most nose bleeds can readily be stopped by firm pressure produced by pinching the nostrils closed for 2 to 5 minutes. The child should be placed in a sitting position, not lying down or with head tilted backward. Parents should try to remain calm and reassure the child, since apprehension will make treatment more difficult. If bleeding restarts, then the pressure should be reapplied for a longer period of time with a pledget of cotton coated with petroleum jelly placed in the nostril.

Rarely a child may have difficulty with blood clotting. The parent should be asked if anybody else in the family has a clotting problem, or if the child also has bleeding from other sites, such as the gums, or has more than the usual number of bruises on his or her body. If there is a negative family history and there is no other bleeding source, then a clotting disorder is virtually ruled out if the nosebleed ceases with conventional treatment. Rarely, nosebleeds are associated with high blood pressure, such as caused by nephritis (bleeding into the kidney).

If the bleeding does not stop after adequate home management, or if there are multiple recurrences, the child should be evaluated in the office for possible cauterization of the vessels. If there is a specific underlying predisposing factor, like allergic rhinitis or dryness secondary to lack of humidity in the home, treatment of the specific problem should eliminate the nosebleeds.

TELEPHONE DECISION GUIDELINES
NOSEBLEED

QUESTION	SEE DOCTOR IF . . .	
1. Name and age of child.		
2. Is nose bleeding now?		
3. Has bleeding stopped?	Unable to stop bleeding, see immediately.	☆☆
4. Was the nose injured?	Yes.	☆
5. Is there bleeding from any other source (gums, urine, bowel movement, bruises on the skin)?	Yes.	☆
6. Does anyone in the family have difficulty clotting?	Yes.	☆
7. Has child had nosebleeds before?	More than three bleeds in the past 48 hrs.	○
8. Are there any other associated symptoms?	Significant symptoms are present.	
9. Does child appear ill or pale?	Yes.	○
10. Does child have any serious chronic medical problem?	Related medical problem is present.	○
Stat ☆☆	**Same Day** ●	
Same Session ASAP ☆	**Appointment (24–72 hrs.)** □	
Same Session ○	**Appointment (4 days or more)** ■	
High priority items are shaded		

ADVICE

Give advice to stop bleeding and have patient call back for follow-up and continued questioning.

- Place child in sitting position, not lying down, and do not tilt head backward.

- Take a washcloth, soak it in ice water, and use it to pinch the nostrils closed for between 3 and 5 min.

- If bleeding recurs, repeat. Place a small pledget of cotton coated with petroleum jelly in the affected nostril.

- Each night, for 1 week, apply a small amount of Vaseline just inside each nostril to prevent crust formation.

- Humidification of child's bedroom when home heating is needed.

Inform parent that child needs an examination to rule out the possibility of a fracture if there was trauma to the nose.

If there have been several bleeds in the past few mos, and no acute problem, advise a future appointment.

CHAPTER **29**

 # **Burn/Sunburn**

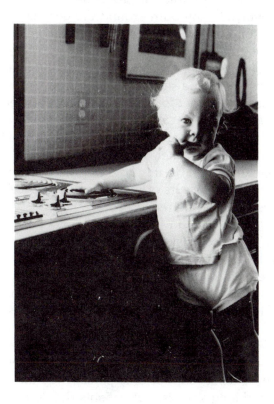

Any patient with a significant burn should be examined as quickly as possible. There are several types of burns. Chemical burns need to be flushed immediately with cold water. They are a problem because the substance can be splashed and scattered onto multiple sites, including the face and eyes. Electrical burns caused by children playing with or biting into live wires can result in extensive damage to the tissues of the mouth and tongue. Thermal burns can be caused by scalding water from a tap, cup, or kettle, or after contact with fire, a hot iron, or prolonged exposure to the sun without adequate protection. Severe sunburn has ruined many a vacation before it has had a chance to start.

A burn should be evaluated in terms of degree, area of the body involved, and its location. A first-degree burn, the least serious, is characterized by redness only and involves the superficial or outermost layer of the skin. Second-degree burns are deeper and cause blistering after the initial redness. Second-degree burns are quite painful. Third-degree burns are the deepest, often look charred, and usually are not as painful because the nerves in the skin are destroyed. Burns on the face, hands, and feet present particular problems in management because of the location involved. Any burn around the genitals or buttocks should raise the suspicion of child abuse, where the circumstances surrounding the burn episode may sound suspicious. It helps greatly to know the family in assessing whether a visit is necessary. If the family is unknown, even mild burns should be seen in the office.

The immediate treatment for all burns is rapid immersion in very cold water. This relieves the pain and decreases the degree of tissue damage. The true extent of a burn may not be initially known, since blistering can start sometime afterward. After the initial treatment, a burn can still become secondarily infected. In this instance, the burn may become more swollen and red. If this occurs or there is any evidence of a discharge or fever, the patient should be rechecked.

Patients with sunburn can be relieved by cool tap water and gentle application of a lubricant, like Vaseline or Nivea Cream. Topical anesthetics like Solarcaine are not advised because they may cause allergic rashes. The best advice for sunburn is to prevent it from occurring with short and gradually increasing exposure to the sun. Initial exposure should be limited to 20 to 30 minutes. Sun screens rather than sun lotions should be used. Infants and young children are particularly susceptible to severe sunburn because of their sensitive skin, and should be positioned in the shade away from the sand and water. Protection from direct sun can be achieved, but only partially, by the use of beach umbrellas, hats, and long sleeves, but patients should also be aware of the dangers of reflected rays from water and sand which can pass through light clothing and under umbrellas.

Following is a chart offering decision guidelines. Questions in the left column correspond to suggested responses in the right column. High priority items are shaded.

BURN/SUNBURN

QUESTION	TO SEE DOCTOR IF . . .	
1. Age and name of child.	All burns should be seen as quickly as possible, if any of the following are true:	
2. How did the burn happen?		
3. Where on body?	On face, hands, or feet.	☆
4. How large an area?	On genitals or buttock.	☆
5. Is child crying or in pain?	Blisters are present in area greater than 2 in.	☆
	Skin is coming off.	☆
	Skin looks charred.	☆
	Suspected child abuse.	☆

Stat	☆☆	**Same Day**	●
Same Session ASAP	☆	**Appointment (24–72 hrs.)**	□
Same Session	○	**Appointment (4 days or more)**	■

High priority items are shaded

ADVICE

Before coming to the office or emergency room (do not delay):

- If it is a chemical burn, remove all contaminated clothing and flush thoroughly with cold water.
- If it is a thermal burn, immediately place the burn site into a container of ice water for 5 to 10 min intermittently, or flush with cold tap water for 10 min.
- If the area cannot be immersed, put a plastic bag with ice on the area intermittently for 10 min.

If the area burned is small (size of a silver dollar), first degree, not in an unusual location, and parents are reliable:

- Advise to soak burn in cold water, observe, and call back in 1 hr. Aspirin or Tylenol may be used for relief of pain.
- No special ointments or creams are necessary.
- Advise that there may be peeling of the skin in 5–7 days.

For the greatest protection, we recommend sunscreen products (not lotions) with a sun protection factor (SPF) of 15 or greater, such as PreSun 15, Blockout, or Super Shade. Also, limit exposure and wear protective clothing.

Section III

Resources and Reference Materials

Evaluation of Telephone System

Evaluation of the telephone system is extremely important. All too often it is neglected until there is a problem or a patient complaint. The purpose of this chapter is to stimulate ideas and suggest practical techniques that might help integrate ongoing assessment of the telephone function into the practice. The most accurate way to assess knowledge and behavior of the staff is listening into a live conversation, which can be accomplished with a double headset or by tape recording. This is not always feasible and also is complicated by the issue of confidentiality.

STAFF EXERCISES

One practical means of making sure the telephone is given equal time with the other components of the practice is to utilize departmental or team meetings for lectures, brainstorming of problems, and informal discussions of telephone medicine topics. The subjects in the Handbook could serve as a guide to the selection of topics or specific symptoms to be added to the agenda of the departmental meeting.

Another effective technique is to role play with staff by setting up mock telephone scenarios with the clinician playing the caller, or two telephone staff alternating roles while others observe and critique. This teaching method has many advantages. It takes very little time and can be accomplished over a coffee break or lunch. It can be a very effective means of strengthening the bond between clinicians and staff. Role playing a recent problem call gives the clinician an opportunity to teach the telephone specialist how he or she would like certain conditions managed, and supplements the written decision guidelines or protocols within the context of a problem-solving discussion. Further, if weaknesses are uncovered in a telephone assistant's base of knowledge about a specific symptom or office procedure, constructive criticism and recommended outside reading can be focused on improvement. Selected, annotated references are provided in this chapter.

Scenarios are included in this chapter for all of the symptoms discussed in Section II. Each is followed by a checklist of important questions that should have been asked by the telephone assistant receiving the mock telephone call based on the Section II decision guidelines specific for a given symptom. A generic assessment form is included to summarize areas of strengths and weaknesses, and to prescribe a specific assignment of reading or listening to tapes as a means to improve.

It is recommended that only one or two subjects be covered at any one time and that you start by scheduling a meeting and giving ample advance notice to your telephone assistant(s) that you would like to get together to discuss how to evaluate the complaint of fever, for example. The assistant could then prepare for the meeting by studying the assigned chapter. Following the training session, future meetings and agendas could then be scheduled on a bi-weekly or monthly basis depending upon how much training is needed for that person's telephone medicine role.

In some settings video-scripts have been created as a teaching tool for groups. This depends upon the availability of sophisticated video equipment and amateur actors, but can be extremely useful for training purposes.

ASSESSMENT SUMMARY FORM FOR STAFF

The purpose of this generic assessment form is to help evaluate telephone management performance. It should be used to supplement each of the symptom specific audits on the following pages. Strengths should be highlighted, as well as those area where improvement may be needed.

1. Was there a four-part verbal handshake (greeting, name, department, and offer of help)?

2. Was telephone style assertive, professional, informed and caring?

3. Were closed and open ended questions used appropriately?

4. Was the decision to advise home management or an office appointment appropriate in this instance? If a visit was advised, was the timing of the visit appropriate (immediate, same session, same day, future appointment)?
IF THIS WAS AN EMERGENCY SCENARIO, WAS IT AC-CURATELY IDENTIFIED AND MANAGED AS SUCH?

5. Were the key, relevant questions asked in obtaining the history?

6. If not, what other questions should have been asked to help evaluate the needs in this patient encounter?

7. Were the instructions given to this patient clear, concise, and accurate?

8. Was the amount of time spent reaching closure appropriate to this problem?

9. What were the strengths exhibited in this telephone encounter?

10. Were there areas in the telephone encounter that might be improved?

11. Are there any recommendations for further study (reading, reference or tapes) or for additional practice?

Section IV

Audit Forms
and
Training Program

AUDIT FORM
FEVER

The mother of a 4-year-old boy calls to report that, on awakening this morning, her son appeared lethargic and glassy-eyed. She took his temperature and it was 102°F, orally.

Were the Following Items Noted?

1. Was there an appropriate greeting and identification?   Yes   No
2. Name and age of child?   Yes   No
3. Duration of fever?   Yes   No
4. Complete review of other systems?   Yes   No
   a. CNS—headache out of proportion to fever? Stiff neck?   Yes   No
   b. ENT—cough, sneezing, sore throat, earache?   Yes   No
   c. Respiratory—breathing difficulty, rapid breathing?   Yes   No
   d. GI—vomiting or diarrhea?   Yes   No
   e. GU—burning or frequency of urination?   Yes   No
   f. Skin—any rash?   Yes   No
5. Are any other members of the family ill with a similar illness?   Yes   No
6. Does child appear particularly ill, irritable, or lethargic?   Yes   No
7. Does child have any other medical condition?   Yes   No
8. What medicine are you now using for treatment (dose and frequency)?   Yes   No

Evaluation: Use Generic Assessment Form on pp. 159–160.

REFERENCES: FEVER

Bayley N, Stolz H: Maturational changes in rectal temperatures of 61 infants from 1 to 36 months. *Child Dev* 1975; 8:195.

This helps the understanding of normal temperature.

Cone TE: Diagnosis and Treatment: Children with fevers. *Pediatrics* 1969; 43:290–293.

"The most important task is to determine the fever's etiology. Once this has been done, therapy becomes less haphazard and the care of the child assumes a more natural course." This article reviews general aspects of body temperature measurement in clinical practice including the process of measurement, what constitutes average or "normal" temperature, and the common and uncommon causes of fever.

Schmitt BD: Fever phobia—Misconceptions of parents about fevers. *Am J Dis Child* 1980; 124:176–181.

The results of a survey of 81 parents bringing their children to a university-based walk-in clinic are reported. An investigation of parent's understanding of fever indicated much misconception about fever. The authors concluded that the great concern of parents about fever is not justified. They coined the term "fever phobia," and urged health education in this area as a part of routine pediatric care.

AUDIT FORM
COLDS AND EARACHE

Mrs. Kelly calls to report that two of her children, Kathy and Edward, have colds. Kathy's cold is rather mild but Edward, who has had cold symptoms for the past few days and seemed to be getting better, was up all last night with an earache.

Were the Following Items Noted?

1.	Was there an appropriate greeting and identification?	Yes	No
2.	Name and age of children?	Yes	No
3.	How long have children had colds?	Yes	No
4.	Were there any associated symptoms?	Yes	No
	• Sore throat?	Yes	No
	• Earache?	Yes	No
	• Fever?	Yes	No
	• Cough?	Yes	No
	• Headache?	Yes	No
5.	Are other members of the family ill with similar symptoms?	Yes	No
6.	Do children have any other illness?	Yes	No
7.	What medication are you now using at home?	Yes	No

Evaluation: Use Generic Assessment Form on pp. 159–160.

REFERENCES: COLDS AND EARACHE

Bridgewater S, Voignier R: A teaching-learning guide for parents. *Pediatr Nursing* September/October 1979; 5:55–58.

> *This is an excellent guide to the home care of children with a cold. It contains a helpful diagram of the ear and clear, common-sense instructions for symptomatic treatment of cold, cough, and earache.*

David SD, Wedgewood RJ: Antibiotic prophylaxis in acute viral respiratory diseases. *Amer J Dis Child* 1965; 109:554.

> *This paper reviews studies of the common cold, measles, and influenza, with a helpful discussion of the rationale for using prophylactic antibiotics. The authors conclude the vast majority of respiratory illness is nonbacterial, antibiotics have no effect on the primary course of viral respiratory diseases, and prophylactic antibiotics have not been shown to prevent bacterial complications.*

Klein JO: Epidemiology, microbiology, and management of otitis media. *Pediatrician* 1979; 8 (Suppl. 1): 10–25.

> *Otitis media is the most frequent problem seen in private practice next to well child care. Approximately 70% of children have had at least one episode, and 25% have had three or more episodes by 2 years of age. This paper reviews recent developments in our understanding of cause and management.*

West S, Brandon B, Stolley P, Rumrill R: A review of antihistamines and the common cold. *Pediatrics* 1981; 56:100–106.

> *This is a literature review of studies that addresses the question, "Do antihistamines prevent or shorten colds and do they relieve symptoms?"*

AUDIT FORM
SORE THROAT

The father of a 6-year-old boy calls in the morning to ask for advice. His son has a sore throat and Dad wants to know if he should send him off to school.

Were the Following Items Noted?

1.	Was there an appropriate greeting and identification?	Yes	No
2.	Name and age of child?	Yes	No
3.	Duration of symptoms?	Yes	No
4.	Presence of swollen glands?	Yes	No
5.	Presence of rash?	Yes	No
6.	Presence of cold symptoms?	Yes	No
7.	Past history of recurrent throat or strep infections?	Yes	No
8.	Presence of a stiff neck?	Yes	No
9.	Is the child acting particularly ill?	Yes	No
10.	Any coexisting chronic illness?	Yes	No
11.	Has patient used home culture technique before?	Yes	No

Evaluation: Use Generic Assessment Form on pp. 159–160.

REFERENCES: SORE THROAT

Breese BB, Disney FA, Talpey WB: The nature of a small pediatric group practice. II The incidence of beta hemolytic streptococcal illness in a private pediatric practice. *Pediatrics* 1966; 38:277–285.

This paper reports the incidence of beta hemolytic streptococcal illness in a small group practice. Streptococcal illness occurred in one child out of 20 and was strongly related to age of the child (between 5–8 years) and season (January–June).

Katz HP, Clancy R: Accuracy of a home throat culture program—a study of parent participation in health care. *Pediatrics* 1974; 53:687–691.

This paper describes how parents can be trained to obtain cultures on their children in lieu of an office visit when streptococcal infection is suspected. Parents performed the culture accurately, and there were no differences in outcome when cultures were done at home compared to children who were seen in the office.

Rosenstein BJ, Markowitz M, Gordis L: Accuracy of throat cultures processed in physicians' offices. *J of Pediatrics* 1970; 76:606–609.

The results of this study indicate that throat cultures can be done very accurately by physicians who have had only brief, informal instruction in bacteriology.

Wannamaker LW: Perplexity and precision in the diagnosis of streptococcal pharyngitis. *Amer J Dis Child* 1972; 124:352–358.

This is another excellent paper showing that on clinical examination it is impossible to predict who will have a streptococcal infection. The presence of exudate, swollen glands, or fever were not associated with any increase in the frequency of streptococcal infections.

AUDIT FORM
COUGH AND WHEEZING

Mrs. Blanchard calls to report that her 6-year-old son has been coughing for the past 2 days. She wants to know if you could prescribe the doctor's preferred cough medicine.

Were the Following Items Noted?

1.	Was there an appropriate greeting and identification?	Yes	No
2.	Name and age of child.	Yes	No
3.	How long has child been coughing?	Yes	No
4.	What is cough like?		
	Dry or loose?	Yes	No
	Productive?	Yes	No
	Does cough awaken child from sleep?	Yes	No
5.	Is child wheezing?	Yes	No
6.	Is there any change in the breathing pattern?	Yes	No
7.	Are there associated symptoms, like chest pain, fever, or cold?	Yes	No
8.	Does child appear ill?	Yes	No
9.	Is there a chronic medical problem?	Yes	No
10.	Are family members ill with similar symptoms?	Yes	No
11.	Is child receiving any medicine now?	Yes	No

Evaluation: Use Generic Assessment Form on pp. 159–160.

REFERENCES: COUGH AND WHEEZING

Bridgewater S, Voignier R: A teaching-learning guide for parents. *Pediatr Nursing* September/October 1979; 5:55–58.

This is an excellent guide to the home care of children with a cold. It contains a helpful diagram of the ear, and clear, commonsense instructions for symptomatic treatment of cold, cough, and earache.

Bye C, Cooper J, et al: Effects of pseudoephedrine and triprolidine, alone and in combination, on symptoms of the common cold. *Br Med J* July 19, 1980; 281:189–190.

Only sneezing and nasal obstruction were improved by the use of treatment. Ten other cold symptoms, including cough, were unaffected.

Falliers C: Pediatric asthma. *Pediatr Consult* 1979; 1:1–8.

This is an excellent review that is very readable. It is available from Pediatric Consult, McNeil Consumer Products Co., 310 Madison Ave., N.Y., N.Y. 10017. New insights are discussed in the management of asthma.

Plaut, TF: Children with Asthma. A Manual for Parents. Second edition. Pedipress, Inc., 125 Red Gate Lane, Amherst, MA 01002. 1988.

This manual is must reading for any parent who has a child with asthma. It covers basic facts, medication, home treatment, peak flow meters, and psychosocial adjustment issues. It contains 269 pages and is extremely useful and well written.

AUDIT FORM
CROUP

A snowstorm has struck. It is early morning and people cannot get out of their homes. The doctor's staff has made it to the office. The doctors will be at the hospital all morning. Scott, the Alexander's 3-year-old son, awoke this morning with a croupy cough that sounded like a foghorn. His temperature is 100.4°F, he is playful, alert, and in no distress. He is hoarse, but taking fluids well. He has had a mild cold for the past 3 days.

Were the Following Items Noted?

1.	Was there an appropriate greeting and identification?	Yes	No
2.	Name and age of child?	Yes	No
3.	How long has croup been present?	Yes	No
4.	Fever present?	Yes	No
5.	Is Scott making a loud noise with each breath?	Yes	No
6.	Is his chest caving in as he breathes?	Yes	No
7.	Is he breathing rapidly at rest?	Yes	No
8.	Does Scott look sick or pale?	Yes	No
9.	Are the lips bluish?	Yes	No
10.	Does Scott look frightened?	Yes	No
11.	Is Scott drooling or having difficulty swallowing?	Yes	No
12.	Has he choked or possibly gotten something stuck in his throat?	Yes	No
13.	Does anyone else have a cold at home?	Yes	No
14.	Is he getting any medication? What kind?	Yes	No
15.	Are there any other associated symptoms?	Yes	No
16.	Does Scott have any chronic medical condition?	Yes	No

Home advice should have been given with instructions to call back if his condition worsened. At 10 A.M. Mrs. Alexander calls back and reports that Scott suddenly is worse. His lips have turned blue and he is agitated.

17. What advice would you now give Mrs. Alexander? (In a snowstorm, the police will go to the home. From there, a trip to the emergency room at the local hospital would be in order, and the family's own physician is already there to examine him.)

Evaluation: Use Generic Assessment Form on pp. 159–160.

REFERENCES: CROUP

Barker G: Current management of croup and epiglottitis. *Pediatr Clin North Am* 1979; 26:565–579.

The two pages describing the clinical features of epiglottitis and viral croup are highly recommended.

Krugman S, Ward R, Katz S: Croup, in *Infectious Diseases of Children*, ed 6. St. Louis, The CV Mosby Company, 1977, pp 248–253.

The differential diagnosis of croup is reviewed and the clinical features of each type clearly presented. Reading the discussion of acute epiglottitis is a must. The diagram of the upper airway in viral croup compared to the normal anatomy is recommended for telephone assistants, but only with the physician's help, as a means of understanding the healthy respect one develops for the potential danger of the illness.

AUDIT FORM
EYE INFECTION

It is springtime and Janie's eyes have started to tear and itch again. She had the same problem last year but her mother cannot find the eye drops she used. Mrs. Sampson calls in and requests a refill on the medication.

Were the Following Items Noted?

1.	Was there an appropriate greeting and identification?	Yes	No
2.	Name and age of child?	Yes	No
3.	How long have eye symptoms been present?	Yes	No
4.	Is the eye painful?	Yes	No
5.	Is there a discharge or crust?	Yes	No
6.	Is the eye swollen?	Yes	No
7.	Was there any eye injury?	Yes	No
8.	Do the eyes itch very much?	Yes	No
9.	Did the doctor see her for the same thing last year?	Yes	No
10.	Did the medication work well?	Yes	No
11.	Are there any associated symptoms (fever, earache, wheezing, headache)?	Yes	No
12.	Does the child appear ill?	Yes	No
13.	Does the child have a sty?	Yes	No

Evaluation: Use Generic Assessment Form on pp. 159–160.

REFERENCES: EYE INFECTION AND INFLAMMATION

Boger WP: The Eye, in *Current Pediatric Therapy*, ed 9. Philadelphia, W.B. Saunders Co., 1980, pp 508–529.

A brief overview of some common eye disorders, including stys.

Mull H: *Atlas of Pediatric Diseases*, Philadelphia, W.B. Saunders Co., 1976, pp 252–255.

Some good pictures are at times more helpful than a lengthy description. This atlas is well suited for the telephone assistant to peruse in its entirety.

AUDIT FORM
DIARRHEA AND VOMITING

The first call of the morning comes from a parent who reports he was up all night with his 3-year-old daughter who was vomiting the "whole night long." The vomiting has stopped but her bowel movement was "pure water."

Were the Following Items Noted?

1.	Was there an appropriate greeting and identification?	Yes	No
2.	Name and age of child?	Yes	No
3.	How long has child had vomiting?	Yes	No
4.	How many times in past 12 to 24 hours?	Yes	No
5.	How long has child had diarrhea?	Yes	No
6.	How many times in past 12 to 24 hours?	Yes	No
7.	Is there blood or mucus in the diarrhea? Blood in vomitus?	Yes	No
8.	Is there any abdominal pain?	Yes	No
9.	Does the child appear unusually ill?	Yes	No
10.	What medications are being used?	Yes	No
11.	What is usual state of health?	Yes	No
12.	Any signs of dehydration? (listless, dry tongue and inner cheek, tears absent when crying, sunken eyeballs, no urine for past 8 to 10 hours).	Yes	No
13.	Any other associated symptoms? (fever, breathing hard or fast, jack-knifing knees to chest with severe cramps, earache, burning or frequency on urination).	Yes	No
14.	Any exposure to similar illness in family or friends?	Yes	No
15.	Any mental confusion?	Yes	No
16.	On a clear liquid diet? For how long?	Yes	No

Evaluation: Use Generic Assessment Form on pp. 159–160.

REFERENCES: DIARRHEA AND VOMITING

Edelman R, Levine M: Acute diarrhea infections in infants: I. Epidemiology, therapy, and prospects for immunoprophylaxis; and II. Bacterial and viral causes. *Hosp Prac*, December, 1979, and January, 1980; pp 97–104.

This comprehensive, up-to-date, two-article review presents the changing face of acute diarrheal infections in infants. Whereas only 25 to 35% of pathogenic organisms were identifiable in the 1960s, newer techniques now permit isolation of specific pathogens in 55 to 85% of diarrhea cases. One of the most common viruses associated with gastroenteritis is rotavirus infection, which has a striking seasonal distribution in the cooler months, November through May. The paper also includes a detailed description of the clinical pictures associated with the bacteria that have been implicated as a cause of infectious diarrhea. These include Shigella, Salmonella, toxigenic and invasive forms of Escherichia coli, Campylobacter fetus, and Yersinia enterocolitica.

Kibel MA: *Vomiting—In Current Pediatric Therapy*, Philadelphia, W.B. Saunders Company, 1980; vol 9, pp 173–178.

A complete review of causes and management. The emphasis is on finding a cause before starting treatment. The discussion covers all age groups.

AUDIT FORM
ABDOMINAL PAIN

Mr. Turner calls about his 9-year-old son who has a stomachache. He was called by the school to come and pick Joseph up because the boy was complaining all morning that his stomach hurt and he vomited once in the health room. Mr. Turner is now home with Joseph and wants to know what to do.

Were the Following Items Noted?

1.	Was there an appropriate greeting and identification?	Yes	No
2.	How long has pain been present?	Yes	No
3.	How severe is the pain? Is the child crying? Is child playing or just lying around?	Yes	No
4.	Where is the pain located? Right side?	Yes	No
5.	Is it constant or does it come and go?	Yes	No
6.	Is it getting better, worse, or is it about the same as when it started?	Yes	No
7.	Was there any accident in which the stomach area was hurt?	Yes	No
8.	Are there any other symptoms?		
	Fever?	Yes	No
	Vomiting?	Yes	No
	Diarrhea?	Yes	No
	Severe cough or difficulty breathing?	Yes	No
	Burning or frequency of urination?	Yes	No
	Constipation?	Yes	No
9.	Are any family members ill with similar symptoms?	Yes	No
10.	Is child acting particularly ill or lethargic?	Yes	No
11.	Has child been seen for this problem in the past?	Yes	No
12.	Is there any chronic medical condition?	Yes	No
13.	Is child taking any medicine now?	Yes	No

Evaluation: Use Generic Assessment Form on pp. 159–160.

REFERENCES: ABDOMINAL PAIN

Dodge JA: Recurrent abdominal pain in children. *Br Med J* 1976; 1:385–87.

A review of abdominal pain with no organic basis. The emphasis is on the emotionally caused syndrome but contains a useful and comprehensive table of physical causes, which are found in only 5 to 10% of cases of recurrent abdominal pain.

Liebman WM: Recurrent abdominal pain in children. *Clin Pediatr* 1978; 17:149–153.

A retrospective survey of 119 patients. The most common socioenvironmental factors found were marital discord, school problems, and perfectionism.

AUDIT FORM
RASHES

In each of the following instances, home advice has been deemed appropriate. For each condition, proceed to help the parent in home management by answering the specific question.

1. A 10-year-old boy has a painful plantar wart. His mother would like to know how the doctor would like it treated.

2. Mrs. Price wants to know what to do for her infant daughter's diaper rash.

3. James has chickenpox. It itches so badly he cannot sleep. His mother calls for advice on how to relieve this symptom.

4. Judy has come back from a hike, and is covered with poison ivy. What should she do?

Were the Following Items Noted?

1. Was there an appropriate greeting and identification?   Yes   No
2. Patient's name, address, and phone number?   Yes   No
3. Treatment of plantar wart with 40% salicylic acid tape?   Yes   No
4. Was the possibility of infection ruled out before recommending treatment for diaper rash, chickenpox, and poison ivy?   Yes   No
5. Home treatment of chickenpox, diaper rash, and poison ivy?   Yes   No

Evaluation: Use Generic Assessment Form on pp. 159–160.

REFERENCES: RASHES

Krugman S, Ward R, Katz S: Varicella-zoster infections, in *Infectious Diseases of Children*, St. Louis, The C.V. Mosby Company, 1977, pp 451–455.

A classical review that is particularly helpful because of the clinical description, pictures, and schematic diagrams depicting the clinical course of the illness.

Krugman S, Ward R, Katz S: Streptococcal infections, group A, including scarlet fever, in *Infectious Diseases of Children*, St. Louis, The C.V. Mosby Company, 1977, pp 340–351.

An excellent clinical description that is a must for those dealing with streptococcal infections.

Levine N: Recognizing and removing warts: New approaches to an age-old affliction. *Modern Medicine* Dec 15–Jan 15, 1981; pp 34–41.

A good up-to-date review.

Wiener F: The relationship of diapers to diaper rashes in the one-month-old infant. *J Pediatr* 1979; 95:422–424.

This study, although not controlled, found cloth diapers superior to pampers and plastic pants in preventing diaper rash.

AUDIT FORM
CHRONIC OR RECURRENT HEADACHE

Mrs. Jones calls to report that her son David has had headaches for the past 6 months. They seemed to be better but now are occurring more often. She thinks it may be related to the stress of school and the pressure of other activities, but she is worried that it could be something physical. She expresses her worry about the possibility of a brain tumor.

Were the Following Items Noted?

1.	Was there an appropriate greeting and identification?	Yes	No
2.	How long have headaches been present?	Yes	No
3.	Are there any associated symptoms: vomiting, stiff neck, vision problems, behavior change, drowsiness, a pattern of early morning vomiting?	Yes	No
4.	Has there been a recent history of head injury?	Yes	No
5.	How often are headaches?	Yes	No
6.	Are they getting worse in intensity?	Yes	No
7.	Does child appear ill?	Yes	No
8.	Are you giving any medication? Is it effective?	Yes	No
9.	Are there any other chronic medical problems?	Yes	No

Evaluation: Use Generic Assessment Form on pp. 159–160.

REFERENCES: HEADACHE

Moe PG: Headaches in children. Meeting the challenge of management. *Postgrad Med* April 1978; 63:169–174.

A readable review of the different types of headache in children. The emphasis is on differential diagnosis and management.

Rothner AD: Headaches in children: A review. *Headache* 1979; 19:156–162.

A review with an emphasis on the clinical history in evaluating the various causes of headache.

AUDIT FORM
BURNING AND FREQUENCY OF URINATION

Mrs. Gilette has just arrived home and found her 8-year-old daughter going to the bathroom every 5 minutes. She cries each time she urinates. The doctor is out for the morning but will be in the office at 2 P.M. The mother would like to know what to do until then.

Were the following items noted?

1.	Was there an appropriate greeting and identification?	Yes	No
2.	Name and age of child?	Yes	No
3.	How long have symptoms been present?	Yes	No
4.	Is there any vaginal redness or discharge?	Yes	No
5.	Is there fever?	Yes	No
6.	Does child appear ill?	Yes	No
7.	Has she had a recent bubble bath?	Yes	No
8.	Is there rectal itching?	Yes	No
9.	Has there been a previous UTI?	Yes	No

Evaluation: Use Generic Assessment Form on pp. 159–160.

REFERENCES: BURNING OR FREQUENCY OF URINATION

Kunin C, DeGroot J, Uehling D, Ramgopal V: Detection of urinary tract infections in 3–5 year old girls by mothers using a nitrite indicator strip. *Pediatrics* 1976; 57:829–835.

This carefully collected data indicates that the Nitrite Strip is an efficient method of detecting urinary tract infections.

Rapkin R: Urinary tract infection in childhood. *Pediatrics* 1977; 60:508–511.

A good basic review article.

Simmons, RJ: Acute vulvovaginitis caused by soap products. *Obstet Gynecol* 1955; 6:447–448.

This paper reports on the bubble bath syndrome in 116 females, and subsequent reports have documented the same symptoms in males.

AUDIT FORM
POISONING

Example 1

A panic-stricken mother calls—Johnny took a whole bottle of aspirin (information not given but to be obtained by the telephone assistant). Johnny is 5 years old, weighs 50 pounds, got into a whole bottle of 25 baby aspirin 5 minutes ago. He is acting well. The dose ingested is 2,000 mg (25 pills × 80 mg) or 80 mg/kg. (There is a syrup of ipecac in the home.)

Example 2

Mrs. Smith arrived home from work and found her 3-year-old acting strangely, and her breath smelled funny—like turpentine. She checked her closets and found a spilled bottle of Old English furniture polish tipped over and open, with the contents spilled onto the floor and shelf.

Were the Following Items Noted?

1. Was there an appropriate greeting and identification?   Yes   No
2. Obtained the patient's name, address, and phone number?   Yes   No
3. Identified the substance ingested?   Yes   No
4. Condition of the child?   Yes   No
5. How long ago was it ingested?   Yes   No
6. Has Poison Control Center been called?   Yes   No
   a) What is their advice?
7. Do you have syrup of ipecac at home?   Yes   No
   (Re: Example #1)
8. Has vomiting already taken place?   Yes   No
9. What are the details of the ingestion?   Yes   No
   a) Nature of substance
   b) Amount ingested
10. What is weight of child? (Re: Example #1)   Yes   No
11. Was the advice appropriate for:
    a) Example 1 (syrup of ipecac)   Yes   No
    b) Example 2 (immediate appointment)   Yes   No
12. Was consultation with the physician obtained and appropriate?   Yes   No
13. Were the instructions for giving the syrup of ipecac in example #1 appropriate, clear, and concise?   Yes   No

REFERENCES: POISONING

Handbook of Common Poisonings in Children. HEW publication no. (FDA) 76–7004. US Department of Health, Education and Welfare, Public Health Service/Food and Drug Administration, 1976.

This small pamphlet (105 pages) prepared by the Food and Drug Administration is an excellent resource.

Pascoe D, Grossman M: *Quick Reference to Pediatric Emergencies*, Philadelphia, JB Lippincott Co, 1973; pp 299–338.

Scherz RG, Latham GH, Stracner CE: Child-resistant containers can prevent poisoning. *Pediatrics* 1969; 43:84–90.

A classical paper on poison prevention.

Evaluation: Use Generic Assessment Form on pp. 159–160.

AUDIT FORM
ANIMAL BITES

Mrs. Goldstein calls the office on Saturday morning. She is very distraught. Her neighbor's dog, a pet they purchased last week, bit their 7-year-old daughter, Becky. The best they can determine is that Becky went to pet the collie and the dog turned on her. Mrs. Goldstein is afraid of rabies and wants to know what to do. (Information not given: Becky's last and fourth tetanus immunization was at age 4 years.)

Were the Following Items Noted?

1.	Was there an appropriate greeting and identification?	Yes	No
2.	Patient's name, address, and phone number?	Yes	No
3.	Immunization status of dog?	Yes	No
4.	Is animal available for observation?	Yes	No
5.	Was attack unprovoked or was animal approached?	Yes	No
6.	Was the skin broken?	Yes	No
7.	Location of bites?	Yes	No
8.	Date of child's last tetanus immunization?	Yes	No

Evaluation: Use Generic Assessment Form on pp. 159–160.

REFERENCES: ANIMAL BITES

Grossman M, Pascoe D: *Quick Reference to Pediatric Emergencies*, Philadelphia, JB Lippincott & Company, 1973, pp 261–3.

A useful reference to keep handy.

Kizer KW: Epidemiologic and clinical aspects of animal bite injuries. *JACEP* 1979: 8:134–41.

An interesting article analyzing data on 307 bites, describing almost anything you would like to know about animal bites. For example, dog bites are twice as common among males, while cat bites and scratches were twice as common among females.

Miller A, Nathanson N: Rabies: Recent advances in pathogenesis and control. *Ann Neurol* 1977; 2:511–19.

This paper reviews the virology, immunology, pathogenesis, treatment, and prophylaxis of rabies in a manner that should be interesting to all providers of health care.

AUDIT FORM
INSECT BITES AND STINGS

1. Mrs. Owens reports that her daughter has been bitten by a spider, and that there is marked swelling around the bite. What advice would you give her?

    Question: a) Home advice or appointment?

    b) If an appointment, would you advise her to do anything before coming to the office, or ask any other questions?

2. Mrs. Brooks calls because Victoria has a tick embedded into the skin just behind the ear. She wants to know whether she should come in and have it removed, or could she do it herself.

    Question: a) Would you advise her to do it herself at home?

    b) What advice would you give her?

3. Mrs. Jamison calls because Thomas, their son, stepped on a bee while walking barefoot to the swimming pool. He is limping because of the pain. Mrs. Jamison is worried because the last time this happened his foot became quite swollen. She wants to know if she should bring Thomas in to see the doctor.

Were the Following Items Noted?

1. Was there an appropriate greeting and identification?   Yes   No
2. Description of the areas of bite—redness, swelling, itchy?   Yes   No
3. Details of the history of previous reaction—local versus generalized? Mild versus severe?   Yes   No
4. Is there any difficulty breathing, light-headedness, swelling around the eyes, or generalized rash?   Yes   No

Evaluation: Use Generic Assessment Form on pp. 159–160.

REFERENCES: INSECT BITES

Bradford WD, Hawkins HK: Rocky Mountain Spotted Fever in childhood. *Am J Dis Child* 1977; 131:1228–1232.

A review of the disease in 138 children. It contains a good deal of medical terminology, but clinical parts are readable.

Snyder C, Temple A: Arthropod bites and strings, in Gells S and Kagan B (eds): *Current Pediatric Therapy*, ed 9. Philadelphia, W.B. Saunders Co, 1980; pp 482–83.

A good basic discussion of bites by the spider, scorpion, bee, fly, and aquatic animal.

Toewe CH: Bug bites and stings. *Am Fam Physician* 1980; 21:90–95.

Excellent comprehensive review.

AUDIT FORM
PUNCTURE WOUNDS, LACERATIONS, AND ABRASIONS

Mrs. Jurgens calls to report that her 10-year-old son stepped on a nail (small tack lying in the field) on the way to the pool. She states that Ralph is in pain and wants to know what to do.

Were the Following Items Noted?

1.	Was there an appropriate greeting and identification?	Yes	No
2.	Name and age of child?	Yes	No
3.	When, where and how injury occurred?	Yes	No
4.	Was nail clean or dirty?	Yes	No
5.	Where on body?	Yes	No
6.	Does wound appear very deep?	Yes	No
7.	Is there foreign material in the wound?	Yes	No
8.	Are there signs of infection (redness, swelling, streaks, or discharge)?	Yes	No
9.	Is there active bleeding?	Yes	No
10.	Is Ralph's tetanus immunization up-to-date?	Yes	No
11.	When was his last booster?	Yes	No

Evaluation: Use Generic Assessment Form on pp. 159–160.

REFERENCES: PUNCTURE WOUNDS, LACERATIONS, AND ABRASIONS

American Academy of Pediatrics. In *Report of the Committee on Infectious Diseases. Tetanus*, ed. 21. Evanston, Illinois, 1988, pp 409–414.

This is an authoritative review of the cause, epidemiology, and treatment of tetanus.

AUDIT FORM
HEAD INJURY

Robert, 7 years old, tripped and hit his head against the wall. He got up right away and, although he feels fine and is acting normally, there is a small bump on his forehead that hurts. His father has called for advice.

Were the Following Items Noted?

1. Was there an appropriate greeting and identification?   Yes   No
2. Name and age of child?   Yes   No
3. When did injury happen?   Yes   No
4. Is child acting normally?   Yes   No
5. Was there any loss of consciousness?   Yes   No
6. Are there any symptoms, such as lethargy, pallor, loss of memory, visual disturbances, mental confusion, or strange behavior?   Yes   No
7. Has there been a serious head injury in the past?   Yes   No
8. Is there any evidence that any other part of the body has been injured?   Yes   No

Evaluation: Use Generic Assessment Form on pp. 159–160.

REFERENCES: HEAD INJURY

McLaurin RL: *Head injury in Current Pediatric Therapy*, ed 9. (Gellis S and Kagan B). Philadelphia, WB Saunders Co, 1980, pp 40–43.

A brief review of classification and management.

Rosman NP: Pediatric head injuries. *Pediatr Ann* 1978; 7:55–74.

A good review with discussion of scalp swellings, fractures, and cerebral concussion.

Singer H, Freeman J: Head trauma for the pediatrician. *Pediatrics* 1978; 62:819–825.

This paper is written for the physician, but it should be of interest to telephone assistants to read about the hospitalized child.

Walleck C: Head Trauma in children. *Nurs Clin North Am.* 1980; 15:115–127.

This is an overview of pediatric head injuries from the nurse's perspective.

AUDIT FORM
STRAINS AND SPRAINS

Max has just come home from his first day of high school soccer practice. His whole body aches. The main problems are a sore thigh muscle and a very slightly sprained ankle. He felt the thigh muscle pull while he was doing wind sprints. As he was leaving practice, he stepped into a gully and felt his ankle twist a little. He did not fall and was able to walk home without too much discomfort. His father just came home from work and found him limping around and called for help.

Were the Following Items Noted?

1.	Was there an appropriate greeting and identification?	Yes	No
2.	Name and age of child?	Yes	No
3.	Description of how injury occurred?	Yes	No
4.	Is pain very severe?	Yes	No
5.	Is there fever?	Yes	No
6.	Does Max appear ill?	Yes	No
7.	Is ankle very swollen, red, or hot?	Yes	No
8.	Is Max in very much pain when ankle is moved?	Yes	No
9.	What home treatment has been done thus far, if any?	Yes	No

Evaluation: Use Generic Assessment Form on pp. 159–160.

REFERENCES: STRAINS AND SPRAINS

DeHaven KE: Athletic injuries in adolescents. *Pediatr Ann* 1978; 7:96–119.

A helpful classification of injuries. The medical discussion is technical, but the classification and statistical discussion is appropriate for telephone assistants.

Zimbler S: Injuries related to sports and recreation in *Current Pediatric Therapy* ed 9. (Gellis S and Kagan B). Philadelphia, WB Saunders Co, 1980, pp 700–703.

A good review.

AUDIT FORM
NOSEBLEEDS

Charles Sullivan is a 7-year-old boy whose mother found blood on his pillowcase when she went to wake him this morning. He was sent home from school this afternoon with another nosebleed. As soon as he got home, it started again. Mrs. Sullivan has never had to stop the bleeding herself. She asks for advice.

Were the Following Items Noted?

1. Was there an appropriate greeting and identification?   Yes   No
2. Name and age of child?   Yes   No
3. Whether bleeding was present now?   Yes   No
4. Is there bleeding from other parts of the body?   Yes   No
5. Is there a family history of a clotting disorder?   Yes   No
6. Has child had nosebleeds in the past?   Yes   No
7. Does child appear ill?   Yes   No
8. Is there any serious underlying chronic medical problem?   Yes   No

Evaluation: Use Generic Assessment Form on pp. 159–160.

REFERENCES: NOSEBLEED

Birrell JF: *The Nasal Vestibule and Septum in Paediatric Otolaryngology,* Chicago, Year Book Medical Publishers, Inc, 1978, pp 58–60.

A general article.

Chason WP: *Epistaxis in Current Pediatric Therapy,* Philadelphia, WB Saunders Co, 1976, pp 107–108.

A brief review of the problem and its management.

AUDIT FORM
BURN/SUNBURN

Mrs. Jamison was making coffee. Her dog got tangled in the cord and knocked over the percolator. Some of the hot water splattered on the baby, who was sitting next to the counter. An area on the baby's chest and abdomen now appear red. The mother wants to know if she should bring the baby into the office.

Were the Following Items Noted?

1.	Was there an appropriate greeting and identification?	Yes	No
2.	Name and age of child?	Yes	No
3.	How did burn happen?	Yes	No
4.	How large an area?	Yes	No
5.	Is child crying or in pain?	Yes	No

Evaluation: Use Generic Assessment Form on pp. 159–160.

REFERENCES: BURN/SUNBURN

Durtschi M, Kohler T, Finley A, Heimbach D: Burn injury in infants and young children. *Surg Gynecol Obstet* 150:651–656, 1980.

This is another survey among 336 children in Seattle, Washington who were admitted to the regional burn center for treatment.

Green MI: A sigh of relief: *The First Aid Handbook for Childhood Emergencies*, New York, Bantam Books, 1977, pp 128–132.

A superior reference book for basic commonsense first-aid for parents and office staff. In addition to burns, the entire spectrum of emergencies is covered with special emphasis on prevention.

Levine N: Sun worship: Reducing the ritual's danger and damage. *Modern Medicine*, June 15–June 30, 1980, pp 37–47.

A primer in office dermatology describing the process of tanning and the various sunscreen products available commercially. .

Pegg S, Gregory J, Hogan P, Mottarelly I, Walker L: Burns in childhood: An epidemiological survey. *Aust NZ J Surg* 1978; 48:365–373.

This is a particularly good survey which describes the problem from a preventive point of view. As in other surveys, the major cause of burns is scalds, mainly in the kitchen. Seventy percent of children in this series were less than 4 years of age.

AUDIT FORM
POTENTIAL PITFALLS

In each of the examples given below, a mother calls in to report symptoms on a day the doctor has been called out of the office for the next 1 hour. You are covering for telephone messages and must decide whether to make special arrangements or advise the parent to wait and see her doctor when she returns. What potentially serious condition(s) should be considered that should not wait, and what specific information in the history makes you suspicious? (Table 9).

1. A 2-year-old boy has been vomiting intermittently for 3 days. There is no fever, abdominal pain, or diarrhea. The mother is now concerned because Timmy seems confused. She called to him and he did not seem to know who he was. He was acting normally a few hours ago.

2. Jimmy fell off his bike and hit his head 2 hours ago. Right after he fell he was a little drowsy, but that cleared up in a few minutes. He seemed all right until just now. His head hurts and he is walking clumsily.

3. Susie is 13 months old and has had diarrhea all day. She has not had much to drink, but has not vomited. Her older brother had a "stomach virus" last week and is now fine. Today, Susie is not playing much, is just lying around, and acts quite listless.

4. Jane is 7 years old and awoke this morning with a stiff neck. Mother thought that she might have just slept on the wrong side, but Jane is quite irritable. Her temperature is 101°F.

5. Claire was just brought home from the nursery 5 days ago. The delivery and nursery course was uneventful, and her physical examination on discharge was normal. Today she was not eating well so Mom took her temperature. It was 103°F.

6. Mrs. Torrence found Michael, her 4-year-old, with an empty bottle of baby aspirin. He is acting fine, but she just wanted to check in to see if there was something she should do.

7. Mrs. Johnson calls to report a rash because it looks peculiar. The rash has tiny pinpoint red dots mixed in with pink blotches. She wants to know if it could be chickenpox because she heard that was going around.

8. Sean is 2 years old. His mother calls to report that he is making a strange sound as he breathes, and started drooling after drinking some water. She thinks he might have a sore throat and wants advice.

9. Tom just came back from playing hockey and complained of a sore groin. Mom called and wants to know if he could have pulled a muscle. Should she bring her son in? He is having difficulty walking.

10. Kathy is 7 years old. Yesterday she vomited once and this morning she refused breakfast. For the past 2 days her stomach hurt and now she is holding her right side. There is no temperature and she does not appear ill.

11. Jim is 10 years old and has had diabetes for 2 years. He was becoming less alert and slightly drowsy. I thought he might be having a low blood sugar reaction and offered him a glass of orange juice. He said he felt fine and pushed his mother away. He still is not entirely alert and I am worried.

12. Tanya is a college freshman. She has a history of food allergy and an epi-pen kit had been prescribed in the past. She calls long distance to report that her right eyelid is beginning to swell and her body feels "funny". There is agitation in her voice as she asks "what should I do"? She can't find her epi-pen kit.

STEP I: Survey of Existing Telephone System

A. Objective

1. To analyze the current telephone system in a detailed, descriptive fashion, including the number of phone calls by hour and day of week. There should be a particular focus on predicting the busiest hours, staffing levels during these hours, and what can be done to reduce volume and smooth out peaks wherever appropriate.

2. To evaluate the telephone behavior of staff and the current training program used to prepare personnel for a telephone medicine responsibility.

B. Methods

1. Use a telephone encounter form to collect the important telephone data (number of calls for advice versus administrative or appointment information, total number of calls hourly and at peak times, number of referrals, and number of same day appointments versus home management advice).

2. Personally listen to the way support staff are answering the telephone and talking to patients (with a double headset for simultaneous listening).

3. Call your office to evaluate the number of rings before the phone is answered, whether and how you were put on "hold," and how the support staff greeted you.

4. Request a representative from the telephone company to observe the telephone behavior of office personnel and the mechanics of your present system, and make recommendations for improvement. This is a service that is usually free of charge.

STEP II: Study of Written Materials by Staff Under The Supervision of a Clinician

A. Objective

1. After study of training material, staff should be able to obtain a relevant medical history and distinguish between:
   a. a true emergency
   b. problems that can be safely managed at home
   c. problems that require an appointment

2. For problems that require an appointment, staff should be able to determine when the appointment is needed:
   a. immediately
   b. as soon as possible

b. as soon as possible
c. same session
d. same day
e. future appointment
3. Staff should be able to present home management advice for specific symptoms accurately, safely, and efficiently.
4. Staff should be aware of how evaluations by telephone are different from face-to-face encounters, and how to avoid potential pitfalls and errors.
5. Staff should appreciate the importance of how the voice creates an image of the practice, and the value of professional telephone behavior to the medical program.

B. **Methods**
1. Staff should read the Handbook and other references.
2. Mock telephone role playing should be incorporated into team meetings where one support staff plays the patient and the other plays the telephone assistant. The scenarios described in the *Handbook* can be used in combination with those created by the staff from actual cases.
3. Lectures and discussions of specific disease entities and management techniques should be regular agenda items for office or team meetings.

STEP III: Direct Observation of Experienced Senior Staff
A. **Objective**
1. To reinforce techniques in history-taking that improve the ability to differentiate between problems that need appointments and those that can be managed safely at home with home treatment advice.
2. To learn how to schedule appointments and keep pace with heavy volume.
3. To learn how to respond to acute emergency situations.
4. To learn how to manage upset or angry patients.
5. To become fully informed about the management of administrative matters, including:
   a. prescription refills
   b. requests for laboratory results
   c. referrals
   d. health education information, such as immunization schedules.

B. **Methods**
1. All new staff should spend approximately 24 hours in direct observation of a senior staff member, divided over a three-month period, listening to telephone conversations on a double headset adjusted for simultaneous listening only.

STEP IV: Evaluation
A. **Objective**
   1. To evaluate the telephone assistants' ability to distinguish between and manage emergency situations, problems that need appointments, and problems that can be safely managed at home with appropriate advice and follow-up.
   2. To improve knowledge and skill by constructive dialogue.
   3. To encourage outside reading and listening to tapes in areas recommended by the supervising clinician.

B. **Methods**
   1. A one-hour appointment should be made for the telephone assistant to meet with each key member of the health care team.
   2. Topics (two or three each) should be divided among the health care team members and distributed in advance to the telephone assistant in preparation for the meeting.
   3. Mock role playing should be incorporated into the evaluation using the audit form from the *Handbook*.
   4. Live tapes of actual telephone scenarios, as well as video scripts if they are available, should be used as springboards for discussion.
   5. Strong points should be congratulated, and further study or tapes should be assigned for those areas needing improvement.

Section V

Appendices

APPENDIX **A**

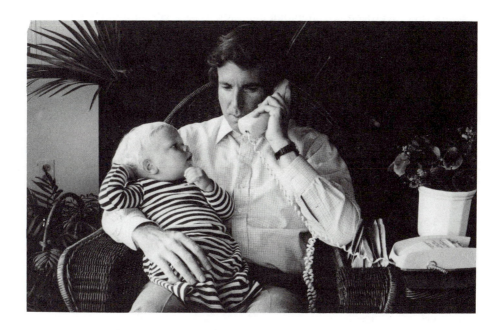 **Potential Pitfalls and Errors to be Avoided in Telephone History Taking**

Errors in diagnosis can occur even when patients are examined by physicians in the office, particularly when the symptoms are mild and the child is seen very early in the course of the disease. The chances of error are increased whenever large numbers of children have to be seen quickly, as in the case of an influenza epidemic. A physician might see hundreds of patients with similar symptoms, thus increasing the probability for a child with a different, more serious illness to slip by unnoticed in the midst of children with identical symptoms caused by the influenza illness. Although these conditions are rare, health care providers can be lulled into

207

Table 9
POTENTIAL DIAGNOSTIC ERRORS AND PITFALLS IN TELEPHONE HISTORY TAKING

Serious Diagnosis that Could be Missed	Benign Condition for Which it Might be Confused	Possible Tip-off— the Critical History
Meningitis	Muscle spasm of neck	Extreme irritability and stiff neck.
Meningococcemia	Benign viral rash	Petechiae (small hemorrhages into the skin) and child appearing ill to parent.
Sepsis/meningitis	Mild URI with fever	Fever under age of 4 mos.
Severe drug overdose	Minimal ingestion	Amount of drug ingested is critical.
Concussion or brain hemorrhage (subdural or epidural)	Minimal head trauma	Changes in behavior, personality, or mood after head trauma.
Dehydration	Mild diarrhea	Lethargy, no tears, and decreased urine output.
Epiglottitis	Mild croup	Fever, irritability, pain on swallowing. Difficulty handling salivation (drooling).
Reye's syndrome	Gastroenteritis	Mental confusion with persistent vomiting (especially if associated with influenza or chickenpox).
Testicular torsion	Pulled groin muscle	Testicular pain or swelling.
Acute appendicitis	Gastroenteritis	Right-sided abdominal pain.
Hypoglycemia (low blood sugar)	Unrelated illness or moodiness	Known diabetes, irrational behavior, drowsiness.
Anaphylaxis	Simple allergic reaction or hives	Difficulty swallowing or breathing; wheezing; generalized swelling; feeling dizzy with hives.
Toxic Shock Syndrome	Gastroenteritis, Diarrhea	Profuse water diarrhea, faint rash, looks ill in teenager.

a sense of false security by the large numbers of patients who have mild complaints. In this instance, it is wise to pause and reflect upon what else a patient could have and not jump to hasty conclusions. This is what is meant by "differential diagnosis." The majority of parents call to present straightforward symptoms of a usually mild illness or problem. Life-threatening problems generally are not obscure. We must always be on the alert and give appointments whenever there is doubt. When the decision is to advise, the door should always be left open for patients to call back if there is a significant change in the child's condition.

The accompanying table is presented to stimulate the maintenance of a heightened index of suspicion on the part of the telephone assistant (Table 9). It presents what serious conditions might potentially be missed, what the condition might be mistaken for, and the critical history, which might be the tip-off that the patient should be seen. The audit exercise in this section is not for the purpose of telephone diagnosis. Rather, it is to raise the index of suspicion and to make the decision to have the patient examined rather than advised, at times requiring special arrangements when the doctor may "not be in." Alternatives include the emergency room, calling 911 or an on-call physician. It is better to be safe than sorry.

APPENDIX **B**

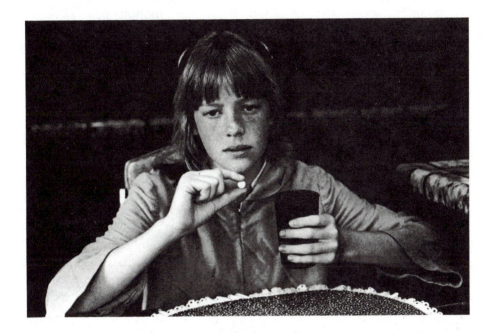

Prescribing Medication Over the Telephone

When medicine is prescribed over the telephone it is vitally important that instructions be clear and accurate to avoid any possibility of error. In addition to advising, it also is necessary to determine

- If the patient is currently taking medication (to avoid excess dosage and adverse mixtures of medicine).
- If the appropriate medication is already in the home.
- If the child has any known drug allergies.

When parents telephone to report an illness, they frequently have begun treatment at home, either with medication or some nonmedicinal home remedy. As part of the history of the present illness the telephone assistant, when it is relevant, should ask if any medication has been given at home (e.g., aspirin for fever), and if so, the dose and whether it is working. In this way, errors in dosages can be determined thereby preventing adverse side effects, and if the parent's therapy is working, it can be encouraged and continued.

The boundaries of acceptable drug prescribing over the telephone should be reviewed carefully by the physician and his or her staff. There is a variety of over-the-counter drugs that should be selected on the basis of efficacy, cost, and safety. Those that have been selected for this manual are nonprescription, over-the-counter medications (Table 10). The drug information was obtained from the manufacturer's recommendations. It is important that all dose schedules included in this manual be carefully reviewed for accuracy, and modified according to individual preference by the supervising physician.

Table 10
OVER-THE-COUNTER DRUGS

Antipyretics/Analgesics: Aspirin

Drug	Strength	Less Than 6 Mo	6 mo–1 Yr	1–2 yrs	2–3 yrs	3–5 yrs	Over 6 yrs
Baby aspirin	1¼ grs or 80 mg/tab	*	*	One	Two	Three or four	*
Adult aspirin	5 grs or 325 mg/tab	*	*	*	*	*	One

or

Acetaminophen (Tylenol, Tempra, Datril, Liquiprin)

Drug	Strength	Less Than 6 Mo	6 mo–1 Yr	1–2 yrs	2–3 yrs	3–5 yrs	Over 6 yrs
Tylenol & Tempra	80 mg/0.8cc	½ dropper 0.4 cc	1 dropper 0.8 cc	1 dropper 0.8 cc	2 droppers 1.6 cc	*	*
Liquiprin Drops	60 mg/1.2 cc	0.6 cc	1.2 cc	1.2 cc	2.4 cc	*	*
Liquid Elixir	120 mg/tsp	*	*	½ tsp	1 tsp	1½ tsp	2 tsp
Chewable Tylenol	80 mg/tab	*	*	One-half to one	One to one-&-a-half	Two	*
Adult tablets	325 mg/tab	*	*	*	*	*	One

- Give medicine every 4 hr until fever is under 101°F.
- Do not give more than the recommended dose (use as prescribed by your doctor).
- Do not sponge with cold water or alcohol.
- Increase the intake of fluids (popsicles, juice, flat sodas, Jell-o water).
- See page 36; possible link between aspirin and Reyes syndrome.

*Not recommended

**Evidence indicates a possible association with Reyes syndrome. The Academy of Pediatrics advises against the use of aspirin for proved or suspected cases of chickenpox and influenza.

212

Decongestant: Sudafed

Drug	Age of Child			
	Under 1 yr	1–5 yrs	6–12 yrs	Over 12 yrs
Sudafed (30 mg/tsp) (30 mg/tab)	Not recommended	½ tsp three times daily	1 tsp three times daily or 1 tab	2 tsp or 2 tab three times daily

Sudafed Syrup (30 mg/5 ml) ½ tsp tid. (1–2 yr)
1 tsp tid. (2–12 yr)
Sudafed Tablets (30 mg/tab) 1–2 tablets tid (over 12 yr)

Antihistamine

Chlor-trimeton Syrup (2 mg/tsp)	Not recommended unless specified by MD	½ tsp three or four times daily	1 tsp three or four times daily	1 tsp or 1 tab three times daily
Chlor-Trimeton Tablets (4 mg/tab)	Not recommended	Not recommended	½ tab every 4–6 hrs	1 tab every 4–6 hrs

Benadryl Elixir (12.5 mg/5 ml) ½ tsp tid (9 mo–2 yrs)
1 tsp tid (2–6 yr)
1–2 tsp qid (6+ yr)

Expectorant

Robitussin	Not recommended	½ tsp three or four times daily	1 tsp three or four times daily	1 or 2 tsp three or four times daily

Dermatologic Preparations

- Calamine lotion (apply as needed to skin).
- 40% salicylic acid plaster (for plantar warts).

Treatment of Plantar Warts With 40% Salicylic Acid Plaster

Apply the plaster after a bath or shower.

Cut the plaster to the exact outline of the wart as visualized. Do not apply the plaster to normal skin.

Plaster will not remain attached to warts on the soles. Cover them with adhesive tape, using a strip of sufficient length to extend up the sides of the feet where it will be firmly attached.

Leave plaster in place for 24 hrs. Remove prior to bath or shower and apply a fresh plaster afterward.

Rub wart briskly with a towel or scrape with a pumice stone to remove upper layer of dead skin.

If skin becomes irritated or uncomfortable, forego treatment for 2 or 3 days.

Do not use plaster if wart appears infected. Call for an appointment.

Parent should not expect wart to be gone in a matter of weeks. Stress that wart might persist for months and that patience is needed.

If any question exists in the mind of the caller, refer call to physician.

- Aveeno oatmeal bath (2 cups added to tepid tub bath).
- Alpha Keri Bath Oil (1 capful to tub bath).
- Nivea Cream (apply as needed to skin once a day).
- PreSun 15 or equivalent, for children who burn easily and need a high degree of protection.
- Sunstick Lip protection (use as lip sunscreen).

Prescription Drugs

Each doctor has his or her own preferred drugs and an individual prescribing pattern. The telephone assistant can be of great help by reinforcing the doctor's instructions; promoting compliance, such as stressing the number of days for antibiotics; and calling in prescriptions to the pharmacy. It is imperative that no errors be made, so the instructions to the pharmacist must be concise, clear, and with the names spelled out if necessary.

Index

217